Getting
Rid of
Gout

Getting Rid of Gout

Second Edition

Bryan Emmerson

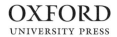

OXFORD
UNIVERSITY PRESS

OXFORD
UNIVERSITY PRESS

253 Normanby Road, South Melbourne, Victoria 3205, Australia

Oxford University Press is a department of the University of Oxford.
It furthers the University's objective of excellence in research, scholarship,
and education by publishing worldwide in

Oxford New York

Auckland Cape Town Dar es Salaam Hong Kong Karachi
Kuala Lumpur Madrid Melbourne Mexico City Nairobi
New Delhi Shanghai Taipei Toronto

With offices in

Argentina Austria Brazil Chile Czech Republic France Greece
Guatemala Hungary Italy Japan Poland Portugal Singapore
South Korea Switzerland Thailand Turkey Ukraine Vietnam

OXFORD is a trade mark of Oxford University Press
in the UK and in certain other countries

National Library of Australia
Cataloguing-in-Publication data:

Emmerson, B. T. (Bryan Thomas), 1929–.
Getting rid of gout: a guide to management and prevention.

2nd ed.
Includes index.
ISBN 0 19 551667 2.

1. Gout. 2. Gout—Treatment. I. Title.

616.3999

Typeset by OUPANZS
Printed through Bookpac Production Services, Singapore

Preface to the First Edition

In the more than thirty years I have been studying the causes and treatment of gout, I have been able to see great improvements in treatment.

We now understand the various factors that contribute to the development of gout in most patients, and, along with this knowledge, we know ways in which the cause can often be corrected, or, if not corrected, can be treated effectively. Why, then, has gout not disappeared? The answer is that there is no magic bullet for gout.

Getting rid of gout requires a commitment to a healthy lifestyle and sometimes appropriate medication. Correction of the cause and treatment to prevent attacks require an understanding of the problem by each gout sufferer, and a commitment to ensure that the cause is corrected or the appropriate treatment is taken.

In this book I have set out to inform all gout sufferers about the factors that contribute to their problem so that, in collaboration with their physician, they can rid themselves of their painful and distressing condition.

Bryan T. Emmerson
1996

Preface to the Second Edition

There has been a steady demand for this book since it was first published, with at least one reprinting each year since 1996. There have also been numerous enquiries about its availability from gout sufferers in many countries and many expressions of satisfaction for the advice it contains.

Readers' comments on the Internet have been persistently favourable, with the wish expressed that this information had been available years ago to patients (and their toes). However, unlike much that one reads on the Internet, the contents of this book are validated and established scientifically.

Although the basic principles of the treatment of gout have not changed, there have been numerous advances in management since the first edition, and these have been incorporated into the new edition. Advice about diet has been expanded and further emphasis placed on the need to bring the serum urate concentration down to less than 0.36 mmol/L or 6 mg/100ml. It must then be kept below this level if further attacks of gout are to be prevented.

May I thank all those who sent expressions of appreciation from all corners of the English-speaking world.

Bryan T. Emmerson
2003

Contents

one

Gout from the earliest times

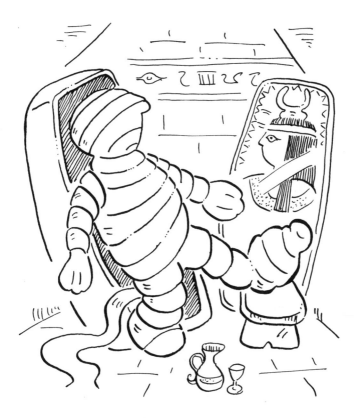

Gout is an ancient disease. The word gout itself is derived from the Latin *gutta* meaning a drop, reflecting the medieval belief that the disease originated with a drop of a noxious humour falling into an affected joint. A similar word is used in most western European languages: French, *goutte*; Italian, *gotta*; German, *gicht*; Spanish, *gota*.

From the time of the Greek physicians of the Hippocratic School in the fourth century BC, gout has been recognised as different from all other forms of arthritis. Some characteristic features of gout are recorded in some of the surviving aphorisms of Hippocrates:

- Eunuchs do not take the gout nor become bald.
- A woman does not take the gout unless her menses be stopped.
- A youth does not get gout before sexual intercourse.
- In gouty affections, inflammation subsides within 40 days.

Hippocrates also recognised that it was a disease that came and went, of remissions and exacerbations.

Gout has an even longer history than this, although not recorded in written form: urate deposits symptomatic of gout have been found in the skeletons of mummies from Upper Egypt.

Like the Greeks, the Romans recognised gout as a specific disease, but they tended to relate it to the particular joint that was affected. Accordingly, they spoke of *podagra* when the acute gout affected the bunion joint (the first metatarsophalangeal joint, where the big toe joins the foot), as *gonagra* when the knee was involved, and so on.

The term 'gouty diathesis', referring to an inherited tendency to gout, was first used by Aretaeus the Cappadocian in the second century AD, who also recognised the frequency with which the great toe was involved and the tendency for complete remissions, of unpredictable length, between the recurrent acute attacks. He also reported that a person with gout had won the Olympic marathon during an interval between his recurrent attacks of gout.

These descriptions are so characteristic and still so typical that there can be no doubt that the ancient writers recognised and were describing the disease we know as gout. However, during the Dark Ages this distinction became clouded, and it was not until the Age of Enlightenment in the seventeenth century that there was any further progress in understanding this disease.

In 1683, the English physician Sydenham published *A Treatise of the Gout*, which was based on his own extensive and personal experience with the disease. He clearly distinguished the acute attacks of gout in the early stages of the disease from the chronic arthritis which persisted in the later stages. At about this time too, in 1679, needle-shaped crystals from a gouty deposit or tophus were seen and drawn by the discoverer of the microscope, Leeuwenhoek. Almost one hundred years later, the chemist Scheele identified uric acid in a renal calculus (kidney stone), and in 1798 Wollaston showed that urate was the major component of the crystals obtained from a tophus. (Urate is a salt of uric acid; both forms occur in the body, but the two forms can be regarded as interchangeable.)

By the middle of the nineteenth century, Garrod had described urate crystals forming on a thread suspended in the plasma of a patient with gout, evidence of high concentrations of urate in the blood. His book *The Nature and Treatment of Gout and Rheumatic Gout*, published first in 1859 and subsequently in many other editions, summarises the knowledge concerning the nature of gout at that time:

> First, in true gout, uric acid, in the form of urate of soda, is invariably present in the blood in abnormal quantities, both prior to and at the period of the seizure, and is essential to its production; but this acid may occasionally exist, at least for a time, in the circulating fluid without the development of inflammatory symptoms, as in cases of lead poisoning. Its mere presence, therefore, does not explain the occurrence of the gouty paroxysm (attack).
>
> Secondly, the investigations detailed in the chapter on the Morbid Anatomy of Gout, prove incontestably that true gouty

inflammation is ALWAYS accompanied with a deposition of urate of soda in the inflamed part.

Thirdly, the deposit is crystalline and interstitial (in the soft tissues) and when once the cartilages and ligamentous structures become infiltrated, remains for a lengthened time, often throughout life.

Fourthly, the deposited urate of soda may be looked upon as the cause, and not the effect, of the gouty inflammation.

Fifthly, the inflammation which occurs in the gouty paroxysm tends to the destruction of the urate of soda in the blood of the inflamed part, and consequently of the system generally.

Sixthly, the kidneys are implicated in gout, probably in its early, and certainly in its chronic stages; and the renal affection, possibly only functional at first, subsequently becomes structural; the urinary secretion is also altered in composition.

Seventhly, the impure state of the blood, arising principally from the presence of urate of soda, is the probable cause of the disturbance which precedes the gouty seizure, and of many of the anomalous symptoms to which sufferers from gout are liable.

Eighthly, the causes which predispose to gout, independently of those connected with individual peculiarity, are either such as produce an increased formation of uric acid in the system, or lead to its retention in the blood.

Ninthly, the causes exciting a gouty fit are those which induce a less alkaline condition of the blood; or which greatly augment, for the time, the formation of uric acid; or such as temporarily check the eliminating power of the kidneys.

Tenthly, in no disease but true gout is there deposition of urate of soda in the inflamed tissues. With regard to the fact enumerated in the first of these propositions, namely, that the blood in gout always contains an abnormal quantity of uric acid during the attacks, sufficient evidence has been already afforded, inasmuch as it has been shown that in fortyseven patients suffering from the disease the blood contained much uric acid, and subsequently to the formation of the table, an examination of the blood of at least a hundred other patients has demonstrated the same truth. That this impregnation occurs prior to an attack is well illustrated in the annexed cases of lead paralysis, in which the patients experienced the first fit of gout when in the hospital.

Modern chemistry has since developed techniques to measure the concentrations of uric acid in the blood and various body fluids precisely.

In 1898, the chemist Fischer worked out the chemical composition of uric acid and showed it to be a compound of the type known as a purine. With our later understanding that the nucleic acids that make up our DNA also consist of purine compounds or bases (and another related type known as pyrimidine bases), the importance of the purine nucleus in uric acid became more readily appreciated.

However, the actual factors which caused a person to develop gout still remained obscure and subject to much speculation, some of which continues to this day. Particularly in Georgian times, at the beginning of the nineteenth century, there was a strong belief that gout was the product of high living. Even Garrod in 1876 wrote: 'Among nations in an uncivilised state, living chiefly on the produce of the chase obtained by personal exertion, or subsisting on the simplest fare, gout, according to the reports of eminent travellers, is entirely unknown; but in our own country, and in many other parts of the civilised world, the case is far otherwise; but not only is gout in its most marked and atypical infestation exceedingly prevalent, but in its lurking and undeveloped forms it is probably still more so, an exercise that has a considerable influence over the character and progress of other disorders.' Thus in many cartoons and caricatures in the Britain of the seventeenth to the nineteenth century, gouty patients were characterised as being obese, gluttonous for meats, and heavy drinkers. Probably the most famous cartoon is that of Bunbury entitled 'Origin of the Gout', in which the victim sits with his well wrapped foot on a hassock and his glass of port beside him, while the devil, with his poker tongs, holds a hot coal from the fire on the painful foot and fans it with his hat. Scudamore describes the symptoms as follows: 'The burning pain of the affected parts is compared to the heat of a red hot iron; the oppressive sense of weight is as if they were covered with a mill stone to which are superadded distressing throbbing with quivering of tendons and spasms of the muscles and the skin feels as if girt with a strong ligature.' Other writers during this period describe extensive adverse effects from gout on the kidneys and the blood vessels. It seems that gout then may have been of a severity and duration greater than anything which is seen today.

The twentieth century has seen major advances in our understanding of gout and of its treatment. The value of colchicine as a preventative agent against acute gout was established by careful comparisons of the frequency of gout in treated and untreated patients. Probenecid, the first drug able to reduce the urate concentrations in the blood and hence remove the cause of the gout, was discovered in 1950 and found to be therapeutically useful and relatively safe. This drug, which acts by increasing the excretion of uric acid by the kidneys, resets the balance point for the serum urate concentration at a level which would not cause gout. The next major development was the discovery of allopurinol in the 1960s. This drug acted to reduce the production of uric acid in the body and thereby reduce urate concentrations by a completely different mechanism.

The availability of drugs to correct the cause of gout has now made gout the most treatable form of arthritis. Moreover, the complications caused by urate crystal deposition in the tissues, with their resultant adverse effects upon tissue and organ function, are now largely preventable. Although the severity of the acute attack of gout is undiminished, acute attacks can now usually be treated rapidly and effectively, and the chronic gouty arthritis described in the seventeenth and nineteenth centuries should now be rare in most developed countries.

two

What is gout?
Acute, recurrent
and chronic gout

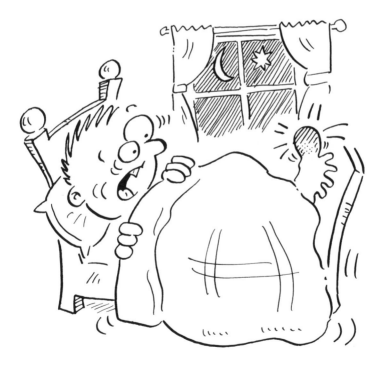

What causes acute attacks of gout?

What symptoms can gout cause?

What causes urate crystals to form in bodily tissues?

Why do urate crystals sometimes cause inflammation?

Crystal formation in the urine—uric acid stones or calculi in the urinary tract?

Do I really have gout or just a high serum urate concentration?

What is gout and what causes acute attacks?

Gout is a condition characterised by severe attacks of inflammation in single joints, which come on suddenly (acutely) and rapidly reach a peak of extremely severe pain and then subside; early attacks ultimately settle completely with no remaining symptoms or disability. Characteristically, a further attack occurs after a variable period, usually of months or years, usually affecting a different joint, particularly of the lower limb.

These attacks of joint inflammation are caused by the response of inflammatory cells to microscopic crystals of sodium urate that form in tissues and joints. Acute joint inflammation with the sudden onset of severe pain, redness, swelling, and local warmth of the affected joint, followed by a complete remission, is so typical of gout that it may provide enough evidence for a diagnosis.

If the gout is not treated, over the years the periods (remissions) between the attacks become shorter and the attacks last longer, settle less completely, and involve more joints. Ultimately longstanding or chronic gout develops with chronic pain and disability, and deposits of sodium urate (tophi) form around affected joints.

An acute attack of gout is triggered by the formation of urate crystals. Urate is present in the blood as a solution of sodium urate; when there is more urate than can stay dissolved in the blood, it is deposited in the tissues in the form of needle-shaped crystals of monosodium urate monohydrate (usually referred to as urate or MSUM crystals). This means the factors that prevent or promote crystal formation are important in determining if there will be an attack of acute gout.

The formation of urate crystals within the body is followed by acute inflammation, similar to the inflammation that occurs in response to invading bacteria. It is this inflammation in response to urate crystal formation within a joint that causes the acute gout. The cells involved are the same as the cells involved in inflammation elsewhere in the body, as in response to bacterial infection. In responding to the formation of crystals or to the presence of bacteria, the cells release a variety of chemical messengers or factors that call up more inflammatory cells and which assist the body's defences against any foreign material. This means that initial attacks of acute gout can be very difficult to distinguish from inflammation within the joints or tissues caused by a bacterial infection (septic arthritis or cellulitis). Crystals do not always cause this inflammatory reponse; the nature of their protein coating may affect the way in which inflammatory cells respond to the crystals.

The basic disorder in gout is thus the formation in tissues of urate crystals, leading to a sudden inflammatory cell response which causes the associated severe acute arthritis.

What symptoms can gout cause?

Acute gout

An acute attack of gout is often so typical that the diagnosis is obvious. Even at the time of Hippocrates, gout could be distinguished from other forms of arthritis because of its characteristic features. One of the best descriptions was made by Sydenham in 1683 and, even now, we can recognise the condition from his description:

> The victim goes to bed and sleeps in good health. About two o'clock in the morning, he is wakened by pain in the great toe; more rarely in the heel, ankle or instep. This pain is like that of a dislocation, and yet the parts feel as if cold water were poured over them. Then follows chills and shivers and a little fever. The pain,

which was at first moderate, becomes more intense. With its intensity the chills and shivers increase. After a time this comes to its full height, accommodating itself to the bones and ligaments of the tarsus and metatarsus. Now it is a violent stretching and tearing of the ligaments—now it is a gnawing pain and now a pressure and tightness. So exquisite and lively meanwhile is the feeling of the part affected, that it cannot bear the weight of bedclothes nor the jar of a person walking in the room. The night is passed in torture, sleeplessness, turning of the part affected, and perpetual change of posture; the tossing about of the body being as incessant as the pain in the tortured joint, and being worse as the fit comes on. Hence the vain effort by change of posture, both in the body and the limb affected, to obtain an abatement of pain.

Even today, it is common for patients to complain that they cannot bear the weight of a sheet on an acutely inflamed gouty foot.

The onset of pain is often extremely rapid and may reach its worst within an hour or two. There are local signs of inflammation in the form of pain, swelling, redness and tenderness. The bunion joint of the foot (first metatarsophalangeal joint) is involved in half of the first attacks. Ninety per cent of first attacks involve only one joint, and usually this is a peripheral (distal) joint, such as those of the toes and feet.

The duration of the attack depends on its severity, with a mild attack settling in a few days but a severe attack persisting for several weeks. Taking anti-inflammatory medication early in the attack will often reduce its duration.

As the attack subsides, the joint gradually returns completely to its former (normal) state and a complete remission of joint inflammation occurs—again, very characteristic of gout. This complete resolution between acute attacks is very unusual in other types of joint disease. Remissions or subsidence may not be complete once gout has become chronic.

During an acute attack, fluid withdrawn from an inflamed joint will show thousands of inflammatory cells together with the characteristic urate crystals.

Gout is seen most frequently in middle-aged males, most of whom are overweight. Patients with gout often have other factors predisposing to urate accumulation in the body. These include obesity, regular alcohol consumption, high blood pressure (hypertension), kidney disease or the consumption of diuretic tablets (usually taken for hypertension or heart disease). The contribution of each of these will be considered later.

Although, as I have emphasised, the diagnosis of acute gout is usually straighforward, in some cases it may be difficult or impossible to separate acute gout from an acute septic arthritis caused by an inflammatory response to bacteria in the joint. In such a situation, it may be necessary to examine fluid withdrawn from the affected joint to decide whether the inflammation is caused by urate crystals or by bacteria.

Sometimes, an acute inflammatory response may occur to other types of crystal that may form within a joint, leading to symptoms similar to acute gout. These inflammatory responses to other crystals (often calcium pyrophosphate, or calcium apatite) have sometimes been called pseudo-gout. They may be distinguished from true gout by identifying the type of crystals. Even acute osteoarthritis, generally regarded as a degenerative damage to the cartilage lining the joints, can make diagnosis difficult.

Recurrent acute gout

After an initial acute attack of gout subsides, further attacks are likely to occur, usually after a long interval without symptoms. The second attack may not occur for one or two years but will almost certainly happen if the causative factors continue, including a high urate concentration in the blood. Recurrences may involve either the same or a different joint. Again they have the characteristic features of sudden onset, extreme severity, and local inflammation, including redness and warmth. After subsidence, a further attack is again likely to occur, but the interval between attacks usually becomes shorter as more acute attacks occur.

Occasionally, the inflammatory response occurs to urate crystals which have been deposited within tendons or bursae, the small cushions of fluid which facilitate movement of one structure, such as a tendon, over another. The commonest bursae affected are on the tip of the elbow (olecranon bursae), between the tendons around the knee, or related to the Achilles tendon (behind the heel), but any other bursa may be affected.

Eventually it's chronic (or long-standing) gout

As more attacks of acute gout occur, remission is likely to be incomplete. The urate crystal deposits within the joints are also likely to damage the cartilage lining of the joints, interfering with joint function and minimising the opportunity for repair between acute attacks. By this time, the patient may be in a state of recurrent acute attacks with very little in the way of remissions. In such a situation, inflammation may only be controlled by the constant consumption of anti-inflammatory drugs which limit the response of the inflammatory cells to the crystals. While this may control symptoms, there remains the risk of an extremely severe attack involving many joints (polyarticular gout) unless the underlying cause of the attack is corrected. At this stage, any doubt concerning the diagnosis can be resolved by taking a sample of the joint fluid (aspiration) and examining it for the presence or absence of urate crystals and inflammatory cells.

Tophaceous gout

Single urate crystals which no longer incite an inflammatory response (see later for the reason) may deposit together to form a solid mass of urate crystals. These deposits may range from as small as a pin head to as large as an egg, i.e. 4–5 cm in diameter. When these are visible to the naked eye, they are referred to as tophi (singular *tophus*). Before visible tophi are formed, smaller urate deposits may accumulate within many tissues. Because of their small size (they are only visible with magnification), these are often referred to as microtophi. Microtophi may also occur around an inflamed joint and, as the inflammation subsides, they may coalesce to form visible tophi. However, most tophi form without any inflammatory response and so cause no pain.

Tophi are rarely seen until a patient has suffered from recurrent gout for ten years. Since we now have available effective treatment to control high urate concentrations, few people with gout remain untreated long enough to develop tophi. However, occasionally the diagnosis of gout may be very difficult and cannot be made before the tophi develop. In addition, some patients have difficulty in taking medication to control the high urate concentrations. In such situations, tophi may still be seen.

Tophi develop mostly in the fingers and toes. However, microtophi or tophi can occur following urate crystal deposition within cartilage at any site. Uncontrolled tophus formation may lead to large tophi in virtually any part of the body. They are common in the cartilage of the ear, but may occur in the spine and have also been recorded within the eye and even within the heart. Their bulk may cause pressure upon nearby structures, such as a tophus in the wrist producing a 'carpal tunnel syndrome' by pressing on the tendons and nerves as they pass from the forearm through the wrist to the hand.

Masses of urate in the tissues appear cream or white, different from normal tissues. They are initially discrete and are completely covered by the skin which, in the early stages, can move over their surface. Eventually, large tophi on the hands or feet may ulcerate, and some ulcerated tophi may become infected. However, once the infection is controlled, discharge usually stops and the ulcerated tophi will heal completely.

Atypical gout

Occasionally gout may be very difficult to diagnose because it does not have the characteristic features. At least 5 per cent of patients ultimately diagnosed with gout do not have the symptoms described. Sometimes the symptoms are only of vague generalised joint pain, whereas in other cases tophi may be the first manifestation of gout without there being any history of previous joint inflammation. Occasionally more than one joint is inflamed at the same time. Occasionally the patient complains of aching joints but there is no sign of local warmth, redness or tenderness of the aching joints.

Whereas typical gout is more common in men, atypical gout occurs more frequently in women. Atypical symptoms are also much more likely in the elderly, in whom gout is often painless with less inflammation. In patients taking anti-inflammatory drugs regularly, the drugs may inhibit the inflammatory cell response to the formation of urate crystals so that the first sign of gout is the development of tophi.

Diagnosis is also difficult in a patient with both osteoarthritis and gout because any one particular joint may show features of both diseases. Inflammation of the distal joints of the fingers (the fingertip joints commonly affected by osteoarthritis) may occasionally be the first sign of this type of gout. In such cases, a firm diagnosis can only be made by demonstrating the presence of urate crystals in the joint fluid or tissues.

What causes urate crystals to form in bodily tissues?

Urate in blood or body fluids is usually dissolved in the form of sodium urate. When it becomes insoluble, it forms needle-shaped crystals of monosodium urate monohydrate (MSUM) between 5 and 25 microns (thousandths of a millimetre) in length. An inflammatory cell of the immune system is between 12 and 15 microns in length. Accordingly, some of the crystals may be longer than the inflammatory cells that may ingest them.

In the change from soluble to insoluble urate, one important variable is the concentration of urate at the site of crystallisation. This concentration may be altered by the action of tissues in certain parts of the kidney, or by water moving from the inside to the outside of a joint cavity, as may occur when the patient is lying down, allowing the urate concentration in the joint fluid to rise. Other important factors include the local concentrations of sodium and calcium ions and the local temperature (hands and feet are often cooler than other parts of the body). All of these factors can be involved in the simple precipitation of any crystal from a solution. However, urate can stay dissolved in plasma and most tissue fluids at concentrations much higher than that which would allow crystals to form in a test-tube. This is interpreted as evidence for additional solubilising protein factors which maintain urate in soluble form within the body and tend to prevent precipitation as crystals.

Ninety-five per cent of people who suffer from acute gout have had high urate concentrations in their blood serum for many years prior to their first acute attack. Hence there is considerable potential for studying the factors which keep urate in solution or convert it to crystalline form. The factors that cause urate to come out of solution will be discussed in more detail in chapter 6.

A separate group of factors determines whether the crystalline urate will, or will not, stimulate an inflammatory response.

Because the human body is so complex, nothing in medicine applies invariably. However, one can work on the basis that crystals are always present in the joint fluid in an acute attack of gout and that, provided an adequate sample can be obtained, urate (MSUM) crystals should be detectable in the joint fluid. Indeed they can sometimes be found in joint fluid between acute attacks when there is no remaining inflammation. Persistent inability to find urate crystals within joint fluid should throw the diagnosis of gout into doubt.

The appearance of the crystals under polarised light is usually sufficiently distinctive for the pathologist to be able to identify the crystal as urate and to differentiate it from other types of crystal (figure 2.1). Identification can be confirmed by adding a device called a red plate compensator to the polariser. This provides characteristic colour changes when a urate crystal is rotated in the polarised light.

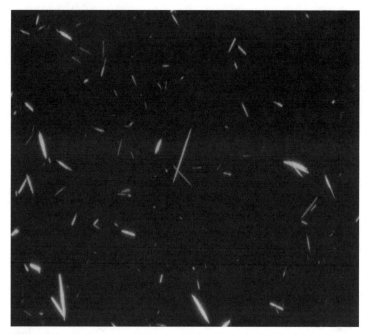

Figure 2.1 Urate crystals photographed under polarised light.

Why do urate crystals sometimes cause inflammation?

Inflammatory cells respond to foreign bodies, principally bacteria, by ingesting them and then digesting them within the cell substance (cytoplasm). Unless they are coated with something (such as a protein) which prevents the inflammatory response, urate crystals in the tissues or joints act as foreign bodies and cause inflammatory cells to be attracted to the site. The inflammatory cells respond to the crystals as if they were bacteria, first ingesting them and then attempting to digest them using enzymes secreted into the cell cavity (vacuole) surrounding the crystals. If the crystal cannot be digested, the cell may rupture and discharge some of these digestive enzymes into the surrounding tissues, aggravating the local inflammation. In addition, the inflammatory cell response leads to the

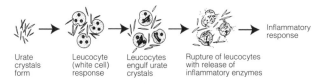

Urate crystals form → Leucocyte (white cell) response → Leucocytes engulf urate crystals → Rupture of leucocytes with release of inflammatory enzymes → Inflammatory response

Figure 2.2 The reaction between urate crystals and white cells (leucocytes) that causes the inflammatory response.

formation of several other local factors which attract other inflammatory cells to respond to the foreign material. These widen the blood vessels, increasing the blood supply, and the tissues are infiltrated further by other inflammatory cells, particularly one type called neutrophil cells. Thus the formation of crystals can attract inflammatory cells which, in the attempt to engulf the crystals, may release a number of inflammatory mediators, or cytokines. Although the inflammatory response is intended to remove the damaging foreign agent, it may result in additional local damage to the tissues (figure 2.2).

The deposition of urate crystals in cartilage often causes no symptoms and does not provoke an inflammatory response. This is due either to the protein coating of the crystal in this site or to a peculiarity of cartilage. As well, the long-term consumption of non-steroidal anti-inflammatory drugs (NSAIDs) may block or reduce the inflammatory response to urate crystal formation. Whatever the explanation, the formation of tophi in some tissues may occur without pain, while in other tissues acute gout develops. As this acute gout subsides, tiny, whitish accumulations may sometimes be seen under the skin and these consist, under the microscope, of urate crystals.

Uric acid stones or calculi in the urinary tract

Much of the urate produced in the body is eliminated in the urine. In the urine, urate is many times more concentrated than in body fluids or serum. Because urine is usually acidic, much of the urate it contains is in the form of uric acid. Thus uric acid deposits (stones or calculi) can occur in patients with high concentrations of uric acid in their urine, particularly if the urine is acidic. Uric acid deposits from urine tend to be shapeless or amorphous, not needle-shaped crystals like the urate that deposits in the body. They can occur within the tubules of the kidney where water is reabsorbed into the body, or in the part of the kidney adjoining the ureter (the kidney pelvis), in the ureter (tube between the kidney and the bladder), or in the urinary bladder.

Up to 10 per cent of patients with gout have had a kidney stone (usually showing up as renal colic with intense loin pain) prior to the first attack of gout. Each year, about one per cent of patients with gout will suffer from an attack of renal colic caused by a uric acid stone in the ureter. Increased uric acid in the urine is also associated with the formation of calcium oxalate calculi. The important difference between these two types of kidney stone is that uric acid stones cannot be seen on a standard X-ray, whereas calcium oxalate stones can. However, uric acid stones can be shown by ultrasound.

Do I really have gout?

The importance of correct diagnosis

There are many many things that can cause a high urate concentration in the blood or serum. While a raised urate concentration is almost always present in gout, many other people who never develop gout may also have a high urate concentration. In some people, urate concentrations may be high for many years before gout develops. Thus, the diagnosis of gout does not depend upon a blood test, although a high blood urate concentration supports a diagnosis of gout. The diagnosis of gout is a clinical one, depending on the patient's description and the findings on examination. If the symptoms are typical and the urate concentration is consistent with gout, gout may be diagnosed; if the symptoms are not typical but a high urate concentration is found, only hyperuricaemia may be diagnosed. Early changes to affected joints do not show up on X-ray, nor do tophi form in the early stages, so they are not often useful in making an early definitive diagnosis. Accordingly, if there is any doubt, as in a patient with atypical gout, fluid should be taken from an affected joint and examined for crystals to establish a firm diagnosis.

Treatment for gout is long term, so it is wise to be certain of the diagnosis at the start. Sometimes this may require lengthy observation or review at the time of an acute attack. A completely characteristic clinical picture may be sufficient to justify long-term preventative treatment without the need to demonstrate urate crystals.

Occasionally, a diagnosis of gout is made at arthroscopy. This occurs when the interior of a joint (often the knee) is being inspected for structural abnormality by an instrument called an arthroscope. The sight of multiple small yellowish nodules on the lining membrane of the joint is usually sufficient to suggest gout and this can be confirmed by a small tissue biopsy. Patients diagnosed in this manner have often not had the classical clinical pattern of acute arthritis with remissions, and have sometimes suffered from a chronic ache in the affected joint.

Summary

- Gout is a clinical syndrome (collection of symptoms) involving recurrent attacks of severe arthritis of sudden onset with complete remissions.
- Acute attacks recur at increasingly short intervals. These result from an inflammatory response to crystals of sodium urate which form because local factors reduce the amount of urate that can stay dissolved.
- Correct diagnosis is essential for effective treatment.
- A high urate concentration in the blood or serum, while almost invariably present, is by itself insufficient evidence on which to base a diagnosis of gout.

three

Urate (or uric acid) in the body

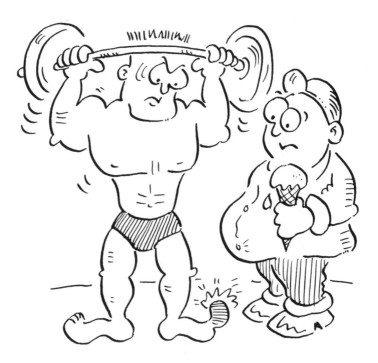

How is it produced?
How is it eliminated?
Why is it there?

This chapter is probably the most difficult to follow. If you have difficulties, I suggest that for now you just read the summary at the end of the chapter (p. 31) and return to read the rest of the chapter at a later time.

Urate and uric acid

Chemically, urate is the salt of uric acid. Urate and uric acid are different forms of the same thing, and which form it occurs in depends on the acidity of the fluid in which it is dissolved. In most body fluids, which are slightly alkaline, urate is in the form of sodium urate. Urate is thus the principal form in the body and is the more correct term. However, in the urine, as it becomes increasingly acid, more is in the form of uric acid. Uric acid is the more commonly used term, but the two terms can be regarded as being interchangeable. Thus the serum or plasma urate concentration has the same meaning as the serum or plasma uric acid. Urate (which is more correct) is used in this book in relation to body fluids. In relation to the urine, however, uric acid is used for the same reason.

In blood, urate is principally present in the plasma and is always measured in the plasma or serum rather than in the whole blood. (The main difference between serum and plasma is that the clotting factors are removed from plasma to give serum.)

What are purines?

You will often find urate referred to as a purine. This refers to its chemical structure, a molecule with two rings, which is of the same type as some essential chemical components of the body.

These purines have two indispensable functions. First, the nucleic acids (DNA and RNA) that control the cell machinery

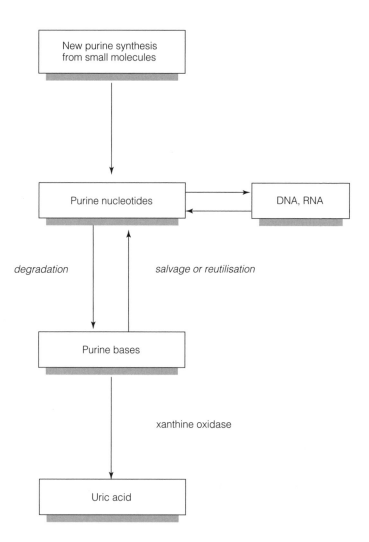

Figure 3.1 How purine nucleotides are produced and degraded to uric acid.

in the body are made up of equal numbers of purine and pyrimidine nucleotides. The purines adenine (Ad) or guanine (G), in the form of adenine monophosphate and guanine monophosphate (AMP and GMP), are thus building blocks of nucleic acid. Any purine bases not used as AMP or GMP are broken down (degraded) to uric acid (figure 3.1).

The purine base adenine has a second function: to provide energy for body functions. Adenine, in the form of adenosine triphosphate (ATP), stores chemical energy and is the main high-energy source for the metabolic processes of cells. The provision of cell energy is vital for the function of all tissues.

Urate is not broken down in human body tissues, although some animals contain an enzyme, uricase, which can degrade urate to form the more soluble substance, allantoin. However, many micro-organisms, such as the bacteria in the colon, can degrade uric acid. This means it is important to avoid bacterial or faecal contamination of the urine if the uric acid content of urine is being measured.

What determines urate concentrations in the body?

The concentration of urate in the body is a balance between the amount which is produced and the amount which is eliminated.

How is urate produced in the body?

Since urate is the end product of purine production, we need to look at the reasons for the existence of purines. As already indicated, purine nucleotides are needed for nucleic acid synthesis and they provide energy for bodily processes.

As shown in figure 3.1, there are two ways in which the body can produce purine nucleotides. The first is by building up the double ring from a number of small molecules (such as formate, several amino acids and bicarbonate). This process of building up a new purine nucleus from many small components requires considerable energy. Purine nucleotides can also be built up by salvaging or reutilising pre-formed purine bases. This is much more efficient, using one-sixth of the energy required for new purine synthesis.

There are four key purine bases, adenine (Ad), guanine (G), hypoxanthine (H) and xanthine (X), although only the Ad and G nucleotides AMP and GMP can be directly incorporated into nucleic acids. However, H can be reused to make Ad and G nucleotides.

As well as being produced, purine nucleotides can be degraded, as shown in figure 3.1. A purine nucleotide consists of a purine base together with a ribose sugar and a phosphate. When the ribose sugar and the phosphate are split from the nucleotide, it is converted into a purine base. Hypoxanthine is one of the major ones. If the production of purine bases, particularly hypoxanthine, exceeds the amount that can be salvaged or reused, they can be broken down to uric acid. Thus uric acid is the end product from breaking down purine bases which are not reutilised for making nucleotides.

The enzyme which degrades the purine base hypoxanthine (H) to xanthine (X) and uric acid is called xanthine oxidase. This enzyme is important in treatment because inhibition of this enzyme by the drug allopurinol can reduce the production of uric acid.

What factors are known to alter urate production?

Body size

A large person will produce more urate than a small person. Muscle bulk is probably more important in determining urate production than the amount of fatty tissue.

Dietary purines—food

Many foods which contain cell nuclei also contain purine nucleotides. When consumed, these are absorbed and digested, some are incorporated into nucleic acids and others are degraded and salvaged. Those purines which are not reused need to be eliminated. Thus, dietary consumption of material which contains cell nuclei, of either animal or plant origin, will contribute to the load of purines being produced within the body.

Nucleic acid turnover

In some diseases of the bone marrow where the bone marrow cells are turning over rapidly (as in leukaemia, lymphomas and other bone marrow malignancies), the rapid breakdown and turnover of cells leads to an increased production of uric acid. This is particularly marked during chemotherapy because the drugs used act by breaking down cancer and other cells. This provides a load of purine nucleotides to the tissues. When these are degraded to uric acid, they comprise a purine load for the body to eliminate.

Disordered enzyme regulation

The balance between new purine production and the salvage of purine bases is regulated by enzymes—small molecules which facilitate and control the rate at which various bodily reactions occur. Some of the activity of the enzymes which control purine synthesis can be altered by inherited changes in the DNA (genetic mutations) so that the optimal control and balance between synthesis and degradation is lost. This results in uncontrolled and usually excessive production of purines and therefore of uric acid.

Increased turnover of adenosine triphosphate (ATP)

As already indicated, the purine adenosine triphosphate (ATP) is one of the providers of high energy for cell processes. In providing this energy, ATP is broken down to adenosine monophosphate (AMP). This can be converted back to ATP. If, however, the conversion of ATP to AMP is too rapid to be reversed, the AMP will be degraded to the purine bases and eventually to hypoxanthine and to uric acid.

Many metabolic processes in the body make it impossible for AMP to be converted back to ATP, so the accumulated AMP is broken down. This is a major factor in determining the amount of urate produced, and can occur in cases of inadequate oxygenation of body tissues (hypoxia), fructose administration, alcohol consumption, exercise, and a fall in tissue acidity. Hypoxia can arise in a wide range of conditions including chronic lung disease but may be able to be corrected by oxygen therapy, as will be discussed later.

It is clear that a wide range of factors determine urate production in any individual at any particular time. Under resting conditions, urate production in a healthy individual must be in balance with the excretion rate. Thus, urate production per day is reflected in the amount of uric acid excreted in the urine over a 24-hour period. Part of this urate production is referred to as endogenous (that is, coming from intrinsic cellular processes) and part as exogenous (coming from the consumption of dietary purines). These can be measured but the measurements are complex and of limited use in practice. Accordingly, in a patient with a uric acid problem who is in a stable state and in whom one can assume that urate production is balanced by urate excretion, the simplest indication of urate production is the measurement of the urinary urate excretion over a 24-hour period.

How is urate eliminated from the body?

About two-thirds of the urate produced each day is eliminated from the body by excretion in the urine. The other one-third passes into the intestine in the intestinal fluid and is broken down and eliminated in the faeces. This means excretion by the kidney is by far the more important route and the ability of the kidney to excrete urate is a vital determinant of the rate of elimination of urate from the body.

Excretion of urate by the kidney

The kidney filters the blood that passes through it and then selectively either reabsorbs various constituents of the filtered fluid (filtrate) or actively passes, by secretion, other body constituents into the filtered fluid to be excreted. The filtration of urate from blood to form a filtrate in the kidney tubules is

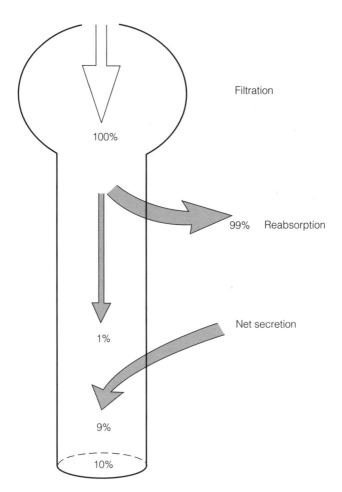

Figure 3.2 The processes involved in the excretion of uric acid by the kidney.

passive (does not require energy), whereas the reabsorption from, and secretion of body constituents into, the tubular fluid are active processes that require energy (figure 3.2). Small filtering mechanisms within the kidney effectively filter all of the urate from the blood serum so that it passes along the tiny kidney tubules. There, the tubular lining cells reabsorb much of the filtered urate and, further down the tubules, pass some of this urate back into the tubular fluid to be eliminated from the body. Normally about 10 per cent of the urate which is filtered is ultimately excreted in the urine.

The ratio of the ability of the kidney to excrete urate to its ability to filter urate, i.e. the fraction of filtered urate which is excreted (the fractional excretion of urate), gives some idea of the ability of a particular individual's kidneys to excrete urate. However, the normal range is wide, between 5 and 15 per cent, with an average of 10 per cent. This means that a person whose kidneys are able to excrete only 5 per cent of the filtered urate is going to have more difficulty eliminating a purine or urate load than a person with a fractional excretion of urate of 15 per cent, i.e. able to excrete 15 per cent of filtered urate. There may be no kidney disease in either person, merely a range of ability to eliminate urate from the body in the urine. Thus, this inherited ability of the kidney to excrete urate is one of the major determinants of the final concentration of urate in the plasma. (The other determinant is the purine load, reflected by the amount of urate produced, as discussed.)

Factors that modify the renal handling of urate include the number of filtering units or glomeruli, the volume of the blood plasma, the urine volume (optimally more than 1 mL per minute), the use of drugs which retain urate in the body (such as frusemide or the thiazide diuretics), and a variety of medical conditions, including hypertension, obesity, and some hormonal disorders, which tend to reduce renal elimination of urate. There are also drugs, to be discussed later, that either reduce the amount of urate reabsorbed or increase the amount actively excreted into the renal tubule.

Elimination of urate by the intestine

Urate is present in all secretions or fluids of the body in varying concentrations. These include the saliva, the gastric juice, the intestinal secretions and the bile. The volume of these secretions, particularly of the intestinal secretions, can be very large, sometimes amounting to 10 litres or more per day, and most of this fluid is reabsorbed. The urate present within these fluids delivers a significant amount of urate into the intestine each day. The amount which passes into the intestine appears to be related to the concentration of urate in the blood and tissues so is greater in the presence of higher blood urate concentrations. Intestinal secretion appears to be passive and not alterable by any drugs or procedures.

As the urate passes from the small intestine into the large intestine or colon, bacteria normally present in the colon degrade the uric acid into small molecules so that no uric acid is present in the faeces.

Assessment of urate excretion

The elimination of urate by the kidneys can be measured easily. All one needs is a timed sample of urine and a sample of blood taken during that period. This permits assessment of both the amount of urate which has been filtered during this time and the amount which has been eliminated in the urine. Most often this measurement is carried out over a 24-hour period.

There is no simple method to measure the urate which is eliminated into the intestine, although it can be calculated by complex research procedures. These involve administering labelled urate to permit determination of the total amount of urate in the body and its rate of production. Since the production must equal excretion when the body is in a stable state, the total elimination of urate can be derived from this and intestinal elimination can be calculated by subtracting the measured renal elimination. This procedure is too complex to be used in most patients, as assessment of the elimination of urate by the kidney usually provides enough information for working out a plan of treatment.

Timed urine uric acid studies

As already indicated, a timed 24-hour urine collection can show the fractional excretion of urate and whether the kidney's function of filtration is completely normal.

Any defect in filtration can be shown by measuring the renal filtration (or glomerular) function. This is undertaken by measuring a different constitutent of the blood and the urine, creatinine, which is fully filtered at the glomerulus and poorly reabsorbed by the tubules. Thus the urate clearance or fractional excretion of urate reflects the overall ability of the kidney to eliminate a urate load, whereas the clearance of creatinine reflects the total filtration function of the kidney.

A timed urine specimen will also give the urine flow rate, which is important because a urine flow rate less than 1 mL per minute (or 1440mL per 24 hours) is less than optimal.

A very high urinary urate excretion can reflect a high rate of urate production which, although rare, is a major hazard for the kidney, and may need to be recognised and treated.

In addition, if the serum and urine urate are studied on a person's normal diet and then again after the elimination of dietary purines, the contribution of the diet to urate production and the serum urate concentration can be determined.

Thus simple studies of timed urine excretion and serum urate concentrations can indicate:

- inherited excessive production of urate
- reduced renal excretion of urate
- intrinsic renal disease, and
- a high dietary consumption of purines.

Each of these can be assessed both indirectly and directly. The findings can identify the cause of abnormalities of urate production and excretion in an individual patient, and reflect the potential for correction. In the average patient with hyperuric-aemia and gout, there may be no to define the nature of the metabolic abnormality. However, in the problem patient or a patient whose gout does not repond to usual therapy, such studies can be of great value in determining the underlying cause and in selecting the most appropriate treatment.

Why do we have urate in our bodies?

Urate serves no known purpose in the body apart from being the end product of the breakdown of purines. Humans experience no adverse effects from low urate concentrations in their tissues. Some people have a defect in reabsorption of urate by their kidneys which results in an extremely low urate concentration in their blood serum (and high concentrations of urate in their urine). These people do not have any apparent adverse effect from their very low serum urate concentrations. One might speculate therefore that urate in body tissues, since it can precipitate as crystals and cause harm, may well do more harm than good. Urate production may simply reflect the amount of the purine base hypoxanthine which is not salvaged for purine nucleotide synthesis.

Recently, there have been suggestions that urate might act as a free radical scavenger, mopping up unstable reactive forms of oxygen that may otherwise harm tissues. However, although this is an attractive theory, there is little firm evidence available as yet to support it.

Summary

- Urate is a breakdown product of DNA and of ATP, a substance needed to produce energy for bodily processes. Urate itself is not broken down within the human body but is excreted, two-thirds in the urine and one-third into the intestine, where it is broken down by bowel bacteria.
- The concentration of urate in bodily tissues, especially the blood plasma or serum, results from a balance between the

amount of urate which is produced and the amount which is eliminated.

- The amount of urate produced each day depends upon the breakdown of nuclear DNA and energy turnover, and these are proportional to body size. The DNA content of the diet also contributes.

- Occasionally, inherited disorders unbalance the body's control mechanisms so that excessive amounts of urate are produced. Although these are relatively rare, they are important causes of over-production of urate.

- The kidneys' ability to excrete urate depends largely upon inherited factors, and the ability to clear urate from the blood and eliminate it in the urine varies. This can be modified by kidney disease, some other diseases, a variety of drugs, and a number of environmental factors, including the urine flow rate.

four

Hyperuricaemia

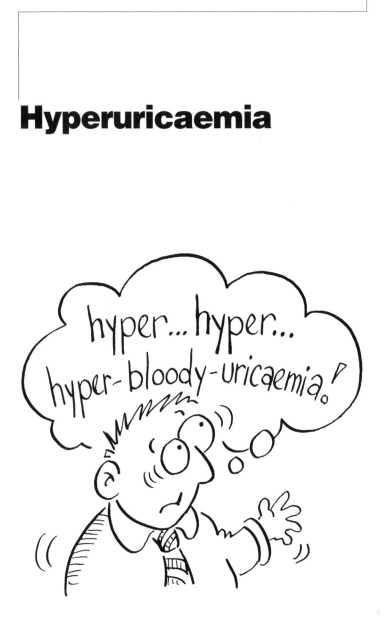

What is hyperuricaemia?
How is it affected by age or sex?
How is it affected by race?

What is hyperuricaemia?

Hyper means high or increased, *uric* refers to uric acid or urate concentrations, and *aemia* refers to the blood. Thus, hyperuricaemia means that the urate concentration in the blood is elevated above normal. In hyperuricaemia, the urate concentration is not just elevated in the blood, it is also elevated in tissue fluid throughout the body, although not inside cells, such as the red blood cells. For this reason, the concentration of urate in body fluids is measured in the blood serum or plasma from which the red cells have been separated. Thus, the urate concentration in the serum (or plasma) is a reflection of the urate concentration throughout the tissue fluids.

The definition of hyperuricaemia implies that the urate concentration is higher than what is regarded as normal. However, it is difficult to define what is normal when a significant proportion of the apparently normal healthy population have urate concentrations which will predispose them to gout at a later time. The situation is similar to that of cholesterol, where the concentration of cholesterol may be high for many years before any complications develop. This problem is resolved for cholesterol by defining as normal or healthy a cholesterol concentration below which the risk of developing vascular disease is very small. But how does one determine what is normal or healthy for urate concentrations?

Definitions of hyperuricaemia

Population distribution of serum urate concentrations

The serum urate concentrations in most populations show a range of values clustered around an average value. However, there are more people with high values than with low values so the distribution in apparently normal subjects is skewed toward the higher values. Thus, urate concentrations form a continuum and people with high urate concentrations do not constitute a small separate abnormal population. The apparently healthy population contains many people who will later develop gout and would thus not be strictly 'normal', but these people cannot be identified in advance as potential gout sufferers. The range of urate concentrations in the population is therefore not very useful in determining what is 'normal'.

Physicochemical definition of hyperuricaemia

Since it is the conversion of urate from soluble to insoluble form that is critical in the development of gout, the definition of the concentration at which this occurs should assist in defining what is normal. However, the concentration at which urate crystals form varies with many local factors, such as local pH (acidity), sodium concentration, temperature, and protein concentrations at the site. Thus it is not possible to define a concentration at which crystals form consistently.

Pragmatic definition of hyperuricaemia

The range of urate concentrations in apparently normal people overlaps with the range of serum urate concentrations in patients who suffer from gout. One can define a concentration at which the overlap between these two distribution curves is at a minimim. This point provides the minimum overlap between normality and abnormality. Thus between 5 and 10 per cent of normal males have serum urate concentrations greater than 0.42 mmol/L (7 mg per 100 mL) whereas less than 1 per cent of people with gout have serum urate concentrations less than this. In addition, the frequency with which gouty arthritis develops rises significantly as the serum urate concentration increases above this value. The risk of developing gout is more than 5 times higher at a serum urate concentration of 0.54 mmol/L (9 mg per 100 mL) than at the serum urate of 0.42 mmol/L (7 mg per 100 mL).

Accordingly, a value of 0.42 mmol/L (7 mg per 100 mL) for men and of 0.36 mmol/L (6 mg per 100 mL) for women has been accepted internationally as the upper limit of normal serum urate. Nonetheless, it is important to remember that these values are arbitrary, even though the choice has been based upon a careful consideration of the evidence. The lower value for women reflects the appreciably lower range in normal women (approximately 0.06 mmol/L or 1 mg per 100 mL less than in men).

This definition of hyperuricaemia implies a level below which the risk of developing acute gout is very small. Its value has been justified over many years by its usefulness in diagnosis and by defining those apparently healthy people at risk of developing gout.

Reference range

Many laboratories measuring urate record a 'reference range' for urate concentrations. This reference range is calculated from the mean (average) and standard deviation (a measure of spread) of the values found in a large group of apparently normal subjects. If the average value in a population increases for any reason, the reference range will also rise. This has been happening for urate in a number of Western countries over the last twenty years, presumably due to lifestyle factors modifying the serum urate concentrations.

These values do not alter the risk of developing gout at a particular urate concentration, and this risk clearly rises as the urate concentration rises beyond 0.42 mmol/L (7 mg per 100 mL). Indeed the steady rise in mean urate concentrations in both Germany and Australia over the last 10 to 20 years has been followed by a steadily increasing incidence of gout. Thus while the reference range is altering, it does not alter the value for the optimal or desirable concentration of urate.

Many studies have confirmed the increased risk of gout with increased concentrations of urate—one study shows a risk of 2 per cent up to a serum urate of 0.42 mmol/L (7 mg per 100 mL), of 12 per cent up to 0.54 mmol/L (9 mg per 100 mL) and 36 per cent for serum urates above this. A large US study in Tecumseh, Michigan, showed that everyone who had serum urate concentrations greater than 9 mg per 100 mL (0.54 mmol/L) developed acute gouty arthritis within a four-year period.

Effect of age on the serum urate concentration

When average serum urate is plotted against age (figure 4.1), two things are immediately apparent. In men, the mean serum urate rises at puberty and stays elevated. In women, the average urate concentration at the menopause rises to a value close

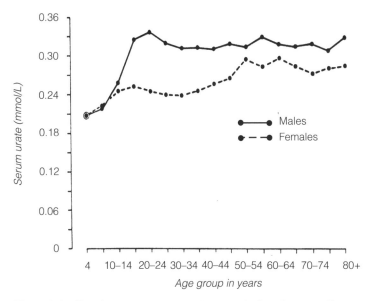

Figure 4.1 How the average serum urate concentration changes with age for males and females.

to the value for men. These differences reflect the effects of the sex hormones on the handling of urate by the kidney. Thus, between the ages of 15 and 45 years, the average urate concentration is 0.06 mmol/L (1 mg per 100 mL) higher in men than in women. This difference is sufficient to explain why men have a much greater risk of gout than women, as has been noted for the last 3000 years. At almost any age, the mean serum urate is slightly higher in men than in women.

Sex distribution of the serum urate

From the frequency with which various serum urate concentrations are seen in an apparently normal population (figure 4.2), it is again apparent that the mean value for men is higher than for women, and also that for both men and women the distribution is skewed towards the upper concentrations. There

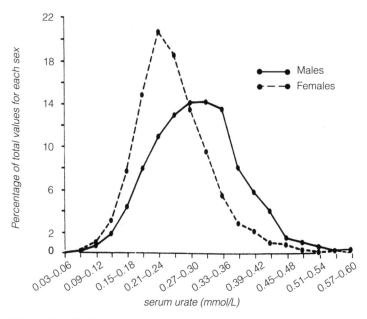

Figure 4.2 Distribution of serum urate concentrations in males and females.

are also fluctuations in the serum urate concentration throughout the 24-hour period, from day to day, and from season to season. There have been reports from the northern hemisphere that the serum urate is higher in the summer, although a similar finding has not been confirmed in Australia.

Hyperuricaemia and race

Many epidemiological studies have been undertaken which look at the range of urate concentrations in populations in various parts of the world. These have ranged from high values in some populations such as the Māori to very low concentrations in some rural areas of England. The frequency of gout in any population reflects the average serum urate concentration in that population. In general, mean serum urate concentrations are higher in urban populations than in rural populations, and the average serum urate concentration in any population increases with increasing sophistication of lifestyle. This probably involves many factors, most of which will be considered subsequently. As we have already noted, the average serum urate concentrations are rising in most developed countries.

For centuries, it has been believed that gout was rare in most races in the Pacific and Asia. In part, this may have been because of lack of access to early records, but many local writers too had considered that gout was rare in most of the indigenous races of Asia and the Pacific. Acute gout is so dramatic that it is unlikely that it would be unnoticed if it were to affect a significant proportion of any population.

The Māori may illustrate this situation. Gout was apparently not a problem with the Pacific Islander ancestors of the Māori. However, to settle in New Zealand, they needed to cross the sea in outrigger boats, a journey that took many weeks. Only those voyagers who had an efficient mechanism for conserving energy could have survived such a long sea voyage. Later, with the adoption of Western eating and drinking customs in New Zealand and the more ready availability of food without the need to expend energy to acquire it, overnutrition could readily result. In a group selected as conservators of energy by their ability to withstand the rigours of an ocean crossing, this could lead to obesity. In addition, the traditional diet of many of the Pacific Island societies was not high in purines, so urate loads would have been low; accordingly, there would be no selection process in favour of efficient renal elimination of urate. With the increased consumption in New Zealand of flesh (all forms of which contain purines), the purine and urate load on the body's elimination mechanism would be considerable. In the absence of centuries of selection for efficient renal urate elimination, many Māori are not equipped to cope with this increased urate load and so hyperuricaemia would often result.

The ability of the kidneys to eliminate urate is an important determinant of the urate concentration in the blood and tissue fluid. In populations with a traditional diet low in purines who have not developed efficient renal elimination, the resting level of urate concentrations will tend to increase in proportion to the consumption of dietary purines, especially if accompanied by alcohol. Thus obesity, diabetes, insulin resistance, and elevation of blood urate and fats are increasingly recognised as acquired problems of many indigenous peoples in the Asia–Pacific region. The problem may also be important elsewhere in the world.

The situation is also exemplified by Filipinos. Filipinos are not usually troubled by gout in their native Philippines, where they usually retain a normal serum urate concentration because they are able to eliminate the urate which is produced from their (relatively low) intake of dietary purines. However, Filipinos settling in the USA commonly have an increase in body weight and this further impairs their kidneys' ability to eliminate urate. They also face an additional purine load from increased consumption of dietary purines and alcohol. Hence hyperuricaemia and gout are much more common in Filipinos in Hawaii and the USA than among native Filipinos in the Philippines.

Comparable data for Japan and China are not available, but there are good reasons to suggest that hyperuricaemia and gout are becoming increasingly common among the Chinese and Japanese as they increasingly consume a more Western diet with its concurrent risks of obesity and diabetes, of hyperuricaemia and gout.

Summary

- 'Normal' urate is most usefully defined as a urate concentration below which there is little risk of gout developing; hyperuricaemia is therefore a urate concentration above this level.
- Urate concentrations in men rise at puberty and stay high; urate levels in women rise after menopause but are typically lower than for men.
- Prevalence of gout is rising in most developed countries. It was not common in most peoples of the Asia–Pacific region living on traditional diets, but becomes common once they switch to a more Western diet.

five

What causes hyperuricaemia?

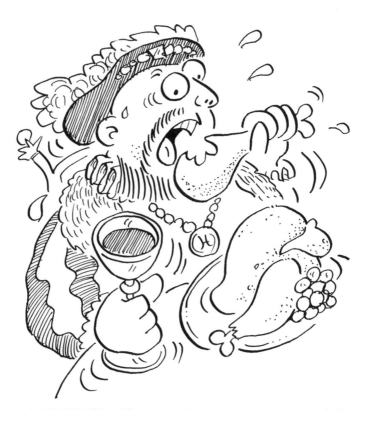

What causes over-production of urate?
What causes under-excretion?
What is the role of kidney disease?
Do diet and alcohol have any influence?
Are other health factors important?

Urate production can be regarded as the load or amount of urate produced by the various metabolic processes in the body. Excretion can be regarded as reflecting the ability of the kidney to eliminate the urate load presented to it. The serum urate concentration thus reflects the balance between production of urate within the body and excretion of urate from the body.

In every patient with gout, a variety of factors contribute to the hyperuricaemia, and different factors contribute in different degrees in different patients. Thus, excessive production of urate will cause hyperuricaemia unless it is compensated by a corresponding increase in the excretion of urate. Alternatively, reduced excretion of urate will cause hyperuricaemia unless there is a compensatory reduction in urate production. An increase in urate production is sometimes referred to as *over-production* of urate, and a reduced excretory capacity for

Table 5.1   Causes of hyperuricaemia

Increased production of urate	Reduced excretion of urate
Genetic	*Genetic*
• excessive production of urate due to defective control mechanisms	• reduced excretion of urate by an otherwise healthy kidney
Acquired	*Acquired*
• high dietary purine intake	• long-standing or reversible kidney disease
• alcohol consumption	• hypertension (raised blood pressure)
• obesity and hyperlipidaemia	• oral diuretic tablets (such as Lasix) and some other drugs
• rapid turnover of bone marrow cells in leukaemia, lymphoma and tumours	• inadequate urine volume
	• increased body acidity due to lactic or ketone acids

urate is sometimes referred to as *under-excretion* of urate. These are the two major mechanisms which result in hyper-uricaemia (table 5.1).

While both over-production and under-excretion of urate can result in hyperuricaemia, each may be modified by both genetic and acquired (environmental) factors.

Genetic over-production of urate

The amount of urate produced each day by the body depends upon the control mechanisms for urate formation (synthesis), and this is controlled by enzymes. Enzymes are produced by the DNA or genetic code, so that small structural abnormalities (mutations) occurring in the genetic code for these enzymes can result in defective enzymes that do not function as well as they should. This may mean control of the body's production of purines and hence of urate is defective, and this can result in excessive production (over-production) of urate.

The major enzyme which, when defective, causes gross over-production of urate is called HPRT (hypoxanthine phos-phoribosyl transferase). The gene or code for this enzyme is located on the X chromosome, and because of this, any defect in this HPRT gene shows up only in males and is transmitted by a female carrier who is herself normal or only very mildly affected. (Females have two X chromosomes, one from each parent, and both copies would have to be faulty for the defect to show up. Males have one X chromosome, from the mother, and a Y chromosome, from the father. This means that there is nothing to correct any errors on their X chromosome. Most defects transmitted on the X chromosome therefore only show up in males.) Thus a man with HPRT deficiency would show urate over-production and might pass on the gene to his daughter. She would not usually develop symptoms, but could transmit the deficiency to her sons.

Although the enzyme deficiency itself is relatively rare, these enzyme mutations can sometimes arise spontaneously and there may be no other members of the family affected. There are about twelve families in Australia known to have this HPRT mutation leading to over-production of urate, but these families include many hundreds of people. There are other rare mutations affecting urate production but they are even less common than the HPRT mutation.

Genetic under-excretion of urate

When the body is in a stable state with a stable serum urate concentration, the amount of urate excreted in any day equals the amount produced during that day.

The ability of the kidneys to clear urate is often referred to as the renal clearance of urate or the urate clearance. This can be measured fairly simply by measuring serum urate and the amount of urate eliminated in the urine in a certain period, typically 24 hours (a timed collection). It can also be related to the amount of urate filtered in the given time period, referred to as the fractional excretion of urate. Many patients with gout show either reduced urate clearance or reduced fractional excretion of urate.

Similar values for the urate clearance (or the fractional excretion of urate) tend to run in families so the average value for any particular family may be lower or higher than for other families. Thus, sometimes, a patient with gout will have a poor ability to eliminate a urate load (urate under-excretion) and a similar deficiency can be shown in his son or his nephew. Identical twins (who have identical genes) have much greater similarity in their renal handling of urate than do non-identical twins (who have slightly different genes). This pattern of renal under-excretion of urate is very common and is probably the most important genetic factor which controls the serum urate concentration.

The range of urate clearance in the population is wide and although the average in a large healthy population is approximately 10 mL per minute, the range is between 5 and 15 mL per minute. Thus, members of a family whose urate clearances were between 5 and 6 mL per minute would have much more difficulty in eliminating a urate load than a family who had inherited a urate clearance of 14 to 15 mL per minute, i.e. who had three times the ability to excrete urate.

This genetic or inherited effect on urate clearance occurs in a kidney which is normal in all other regards. All other aspects of kidney function may be excellent, and even a urate load can be eliminated provided there is a corresponding increase in the concentration of the serum urate.

Effect of reduced kidney function and/or disease

The ability of the kidney to eliminate urate is reduced by any abnormality of the kidney in the form of a primary kidney disease. However, kidney disease also reduces the ability of the kidney to perform all its other excretory and regulatory functions.

Some of the early features of kidney disease are the presence of protein or blood in the urine, or the inability of the kidney to concentrate urine so that urine is passed more frequently. In some cases kidney disease may only be recognised by an increased concentration in the blood of urea or creatinine, two other substances which are eliminated by the kidney.

Primary kidney disease reduces the excretion of all substances eliminated by the kidney, so their concentration in the body will rise. This will include some elevation of the serum urate concentration, with some varieties of kidney disease having a greater effect than others. Whether kidney disease will produce actual hyperuricaemia will depend in part upon the serum urate concentration prior to the development of the kidney disease. If the original serum urate was low and there was only a modest rise with the kidney disease, the serum urate may remain within the normal range. If, however, the original serum urate was toward the upper limit of normal, kidney disease may push the serum urate into the hyperuricaemic range.

Some of the factors causing kidney disease are reversible and if kidney function returns to normal the hyperuricaemia may revert to its former level. Nonetheless, it is important to remember that kidney disease and the kidney's ability to excrete urate is only one factor in determining the serum urate concentration.

Some of the varieties of kidney disease which tend to produce a disproportionate degree of hyperuricaemia include kidney disease due to childhood lead poisoning, kidney disease due to excessive consumption of analgesics, and polycystic kidney disease.

Effect of body weight

All studies into the differences in urate concentrations between different individuals and different populations have confirmed that, whatever index is used, body weight is the most important determinant of the serum urate concentration. However, there is some disagreement as to which aspect of body weight is the most important. Is it the bulk of the muscle? Is it the lean body mass? To what extent do fat stores contribute? Is weight gain after maturity important, or is it best expressed as a measure of weight for a particular height? All of these measures have in common the patient's body weight and, whichever adaptation or modification of body weight is used, weight always comes out as the top determinant of the serum urate concentration. This seems to apply to all races; for example, Japanese school children between the ages of 13 and 18 show the same high correlation between body weight and serum urate concentration as is found in Caucasian races. However, a high correlation between two things does not mean that there is a cause and effect relationship between them and it may be that they are both secondary to something else. So how could body weight have such a major role in determining the serum urate concentration?

Studies of urate production and excretion in obese people and in the same people after they have lost weight suggest strongly that there are several different mechanisms involved. When obese people lose weight, the ability of their kidneys to eliminate urate improves, and this seems to be the main mechanism. However, some also show a reduction in urate production and a reduction in the severity of high blood pressure (hypertension), and this would also facilitate kidney excretion of urate. Thus weight loss reduces the production of urate and also improves renal elimination of urate, thereby giving a two-pronged attack on any associated hyperuricaemia. Another factor may be the extent to which ATP breakdown in muscle contributes to urate production in muscular patients whose high body weight is due to a high muscle mass.

Effect of diet

Diet contributes to the serum urate concentration in many ways, so we need to examine the extent of its contribution and what components of the diet are involved.

As we saw in chapter 3, breakdown of cell nuclei in the body leads to the production of purine nucleotides and bases, some of which can be reutilised and some of which are degraded to uric acid.

Purines in the diet also contribute to the uric acid produced in the body. The components of the diet which contain purines are those which contain nuclei, of either animal or plant origin (tables 5.2 and 5.3). All flesh contains nuclei, and in some flesh foods such as the liver or kidney, these nuclei are more concentrated than in other tissues such as fibrous tissue or tendons. In plants, rapidly growing tissues synthesise nucleoproteins which can be degraded to purine nucleotides and thence to urate. In this way, rapidly growing plants such as beans, peas and pulses can contribute significantly to the purine load from the diet. Dieticians can asses the purine content of any food by the proportion of it which contains nuclear material as opposed to the cytoplasm or non-nuclear constituents. Tea and coffee do not affect urate concentrations, although it may be desirable to withdraw them temporarily during a test.

However, it is not merely the concentration of purines in a food which determines the urate load but also the amount of the food consumed. Accordingly, a large amount of a food containing a low or moderate concentration of purines may provide a greater purine load for excretion than a small amount of a food with a high purine concentration. Thus, the purine load from the diet ultimately depends on both the amount of the food taken and its purine concentration.

In addition, some foods that do not contain much purine themselves are metabolised by processes that produce purines. As we saw in chapter 3, when ATP breaks down to produce AMP and provide energy, the AMP can be converted back to ATP or be broken down further to produce urate. Some dietary components also break down ATP, producing AMP which, if not converted back to ATP, is rapidly degraded to urate. One of the dietary components which does this if ingested in large amounts is the fruit sugar fructose. Despite this, most fruits are low in purine content and do not induce much breakdown of ATP. Alcohol increases urate production by a similar mechanism.

How great is the effect which purine restriction produces?

If most of the high purine foods such as flesh, organ meats, beans, peas and pulses and high fructose foods plus alcohol (see tables 5.2 and 5.3) are eliminated from a normal diet, the serum urate concentration will fall significantly and so will the amount of urate excreted. Purine restriction for 5 to 7 days usually produces a fall in the serum urate concentration of 0.06 mmol/L (1 mg per 100 mL) in people who consume a moderate amount of purines. For someone who consumes a large amount of purines, purine restriction will produce an even greater fall in the serum urate, and a person with only a modest dietary purine consumption will have a smaller fall in the serum urate.

It takes a week for the effect of dietary purines to show up fully, but some idea of the contribution of dietary purines to a particular person's hyperuricaemia can be gauged by observing the amount of fall which occurs in the serum urate and the urinary urate excretion during a period without dietary purine.

Table 5.2 Foods high in purines

All meats, all flesh and poultry
All fish and seafood, including sardines, herrings, anchovies, and shellfish
Organ meats such as liver, kidney, heart, sweetbreads and brains
Meat extracts, gravies, Marmite
Yeast and yeast products Vegemite
Beans, peas, lentils, spinach
Asparagus, cauliflower, mushrooms
Beer, alcohol, wines

Table 5.3 Foods low to moderate in purines

Refined cereal products such as bread, pastry, arrowroot, sago and cakes
Cornflakes, Rice Bubbles
Milk and milk products, plain cheeses
Eggs, ice-cream
Sugars and sweets, jams
Butter, polyunsaturated margarine, fats of all kinds
Fruits of all kinds, including preserved fruit
Lettuce, tomato, cabbage, potato, carrots
Other vegetables except those listed as high purine foods
Nuts, peanut butter
Cream or vegetable soup made with allowed vegetables without meat stock
Beverages such as water, fruit juice, cordials and carbonated drinks

This provides an indication of the extent of the benefit that might be achieved by modifying the diet.

It should not be necessary to restrict dietary purines in a patient with hyperuricaemia unless the person's diet had been unusually high in purines. A moderate purine consumption should not need to be altered. In general, it is neither necessary nor feasible to advise a person to continue a low purine diet for a prolonged period. The purine content of a prudent diet, as recommended by the National Heart Foundation, is probably satisfactory for most patients with hyperuricaemia or gout. Therefore, although dietary purines can contribute to hyperuricaemia, there is little justification for continuing a low purine diet for more than a short period.

The role of diet in gout

It is important therefore for patients with gout to have enough background information to be able to select appropriate foods in their diet.

The serum urate level is only partly dependent upon dietary purines and the total elimination of purines from the diet would usually cause a drop in the serum urate concentrations of only about 15 per cent, equivalent to about 0.06 mmol/L (1 mg per 100 ml). This is not usually sufficient by itself to convert the serum urate from a level which will promote gout to one which will not promote gout. However:

- all manoeuvres to reduce the serum urate will help reduce the risk of gout
- taking more purines than necessary will do the opposite.

The diet of a gout sufferer needs to be directed at correcting more than the gout. Thus any associated overweight or abnormalities of serum cholesterol and triglycerides may become more important determinants of the patient's risk of vascular disease and longevity than the gout. Their management may need to take priority.

Remember that carbohydrates (sugars, breads, pastries) yield 4 calories per gram; protein (meat and egg white) yields 4 calories per gram; fats yield 9 calories per gram and alcohol 7 calories per gram. However, foods are rarely pure carbohydrate, or pure protein, or pure fat and are usually a mixture of varying portions of the three. A basically healthy diet must be chosen in which particular emphasis is placed on meeting individual needs. Usually this is a low fat diet with saturated fats replaced by unsaturated fats.

Fibre and food bulk are important and fruit and vegetables need to be consumed regularly. Purines come from the nuclei of cells and these involve not only animal cells, but also nuclei from plant cells. Thus rapidly growing plants such as asparagus, peas, beans, lentils, mushrooms and spinach all have a high purine content, even though they have other beneficial components such as fibre and minerals. Thus, a vegetarian diet can still be one that is high in purine.

The amount of purines consumed in the diet depends not only on the purine content per unit weight (gram) of each food constituent but also upon the amount and number of grams consumed. Thus, 100 grams of a low purine food may contain more purine than 20 grams of a high purine food.

The diet should contain adequate vitamins and minerals but any balanced diet should provide these; there should be no need for dietary or antioxidant supplements.

The importance of adequate fluids and minimal alcohol needs to be constantly remembered.

Diet must be tolerable if it is to be life-long. Dietary restrictions of purines would need to be moderately severe if it were to be the sole means of controlling hyperuricaemia. However, if one is not able to continue dietary modifications permanently, it is probably better not to depend upon the diet solely to control hyperuricaemia and gout, but rather to have assistance from medication.

Certain foods may precipitate acute gout in some gout sufferers, and particular dietary constituents may precipitate acute gout each time they are taken. Such predictability suggests a specific reaction on the part of the particular gout sufferer and if this is detected, such a dietary component should be eliminated from the diet. This has even been reported with injections of vitamin B12. However, such advice is usually specific to an individual and not transferable to another. Such reactions are only rarely predictable.

Effect of alcohol on serum urate concentrations

Garrod in 1863 wrote 'There is no truth in medicine better established than that the use of fermented or alcoholic liquors is the most powerful of all the predisposing causes of gout.'

Yet, in the 1960s, there was a strong body of scientific opinion which held that alcohol had very little effect upon the serum urate and was not a major contributor to the development of gout. This was exemplified by the following comment about gout by A. P. Herbert in *Punch*.

> *At last the happy truth is out—*
> *Port wine is not the cause of gout;*
> *Far more responsible for pain*
> *Are kidneys, liver, sweetbread, brain—*
> *The clubman should by any means*
> *Avoid anchovies and sardines,*
> *And citizens of every sort*
> *Owe some apology to Port!*

What is the current evidence about alcohol?

After body weight, the extent of alcohol consumption has the strongest correlation with the level of the serum urate concentration. Measurement of the serum urate and alcohol consumption in identical twins with different levels of alcohol consumption shows a significantly higher serum urate in the high-alcohol group than in the low-alcohol group. This confirms that there is a clear association between even moderate alcohol consumption and hyperuricaemia, even when hereditary and early environmental factors are minimised. Additionally, large population studies have shown much higher than average urate concentrations in regular drinkers who take more than 20 g of alcohol (two standard drinks) per day than in those who take less than this amount. Further studies have shown significant falls in the serum urate concentration and urinary urate concentration in subjects who stop drinking. Likewise, studies of serum and urine urate concentrations in volunteers given an increasing amount of alcohol to consume showed that the alcohol consumption progressively caused a rise in the serum urate concentration.

The extent of the effect on the serum urate concentration relates to the amount of alcohol which is consumed. For instance, a large amount of alcohol (as in an alcoholic binge) causes a much greater degree of hyperuricaemia than a moderate amount of alcohol. Even a completely normal person can become severely hyperuricaemic after an alcoholic binge. Thus there is strong evidence that the consumption of alcohol causes a significant rise in the serum urate concentration and that the degree of the elevation relates to the amount of alcohol consumed.

What is the mechanism by which alcohol causes hyperuricaemia?

The first mechanism is that the metabolism of alcohol leads to an increase in the production of urate. During its metabolism, alcohol degrades ATP to AMP which, if it cannot be rapidly converted back to ATP, is degraded to urate. Thus, the greater the consumption of alcohol, the greater the production of urate.

Second, in the metabolism of alcohol, pyruvate, another bodily component, is metabolised to lactate and lactate reduces the elimination of urate by the kidney. Thus, at least transiently and particularly in an alcoholic binge, production of lactate increases, and this reduces renal excretion of urate.

The third aspect is that patients who consume large or regular amounts of alcohol are often overweight, so that the associated obesity (due to the kilojoules in the alcohol) will have its own effect in causing hyperuricaemia. High blood fats in the form of high triglycerides (hypertriglyceridaemia) may also contribute.

The final mechanism whereby alcohol can contribute to hyperuricaemia relates to the purine content of the alcoholic beverage. Beer contains the purine guanosine, which may be degraded to urate. However, this applies only to beer and not to other alcoholic beverages.

Thus there are at least four mechanisms whereby alcohol consumption can contribute to hyperuricaemia.

How important is the nature of the alcoholic beverage consumed?

Is port worse than other wine? Is beer worse than whisky? Many alcoholic beverages have other components in addition to alcohol, and it is possible that these other components might trigger gout by mechanisms that do not alter the urate concentration. Certainly some people notice a variety of environmental factors or activities which can trigger acute attacks of gout but which do not have any known effect on the urate concentration. There has been little scientific study of many of these triggering factors, but they do not seem to trigger gout unless the person is hyperuricaemic in the first place and presumably has the susceptibility to develop an acute attack of gout.

Although alcohol consumption is a major contributor to hyperuricaemia, this does not mean that total abstinence is essential to control gout. A person on treatment for gout who has a normal serum urate and whose serum urate concentration is well controlled should be able to take alcohol in moderation without any problem.

Hyperuricaemia and hyperlipidaemia

Hyper means increased, *lipid* refers to fats, and *aemia* means blood, so hyperlipidaemia means an increased concentration of fats in the blood. The blood fats referred to are mainly cholesterol (in its various types) and the triglycerides (which are made up of glycerol and fatty acids). Raised triglyceride concentrations are not as important a factor in causing heart and vascular disease as high cholesterol.

In general, patients with gout do not have higher cholesterol concentrations than patients with other diseases. However, half the Australian patients with gout have hypertriglyceridaemia (the other part of hyperlipidaemia), and a similar proportion can be found in the other Western societies with sophisticated lifestyles.

As with weight and alcohol consumption, serum triglyceride is one factor which is often correlated with the serum urate concentration. As the most important causes of high serum triglyceride are obesity and alcohol consumption, it is possible that these two factors, which themselves can raise the serum urate concentration, may be the cause of the raised triglyceride concentration. Hypertriglyceridaemia may well be a passive bystander to the gout, but an active contributor to any associated vascular disease (figure 5.1).

Raised triglycerides may also be found in some diseases (such as myxoedema (hypothyroidism), diabetes and some kidney diseases), and there is an uncommon inherited condition in which inherited hypertriglyceridaemia is associated with hyperuricaemia without obesity or regular alcohol consumption.

Perhaps more important than whether hyperlipidaemia causes gout is the fact that both hypertriglyceridaemia and

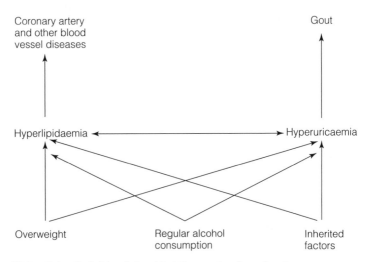

Figure 5.1 Probable relationship between elevation of urate concentrations and elevation of blood lipids.

hyperuricaemia may be manifestations of insulin resistance, which is often associated with impaired glucose tolerance and Type II diabetes and with cardiovascular disease. Insulin resistance is also increased when the obesity is abdominal (i.e. mainly around the waist). Thus, hypertriglyceridaemia in patients with gout should be looked upon as a secondary phenomenon to be treated on its own merits rather than as part of the gout. However, correction of the cause of hypertriglyceridaemia may sometimes correct the hyperuricaemia.

Effect of raised blood pressure (hypertension)

Hypertension is another name for high blood pressure (*hyper* increased; *tension* pressure in the arteries). Some hypertension is due to kidney disease and, in such cases, the kidney disease can cause hyperuricaemia, as already discussed. In the more common variety of hypertension, referred to as essential hypertension, the high blood pressure itself is the primary problem and is not the result of disease in the kidneys or elsewhere. However, essential hypertension may reduce the kidney's ability to eliminate urate. Thus, hyperuricaemia due to renal under-excretion of urate may be a consequence of primary essential hypertension.

In addition, thiazide diuretics, such as chlorothiazide (Chlotride) or frusemide (Lasix), are often used to treat hypertension and these drugs **always** lead to the development of hyperuricaemia as a side-effect.

A number of body metabolites which act on the kidney can reduce its ability to eliminate urate. Important among these is the hormone angiotensin, which is involved in causing hypertension. The newly developed ACE (angiotensin converting enzyme) inhibitors (such as Captopril and Enalapril), which reduce the production of angiotensin, are often very valuable in the treatment of hypertension, and control of hypertension will often cause a reduction in serum urate concentrations.

The effect of drugs on serum urate concentration

The production of urate can be increased by drugs used in cancer chemotherapy. Such drugs cause destruction of cells and breakdown of nucleoprotein from the cell nuclei, thereby promoting hyperuricaemia.

Other drugs affect the renal handling of urate directly. Some drugs act only on the excretion of urate by the kidney. Those which increase the excretion of urate by the kidney are referred to as uricosuric drugs. Other drugs act on the kidney transport of urate to reduce its urate excretion. These drugs include aspirin in low dosage (4–6 tablets/day), the antituberculous agents pyrazinamide and ethambutol, and nicotinic acid.

Something of a paradox exists in that some drugs may reduce the renal elimination of urate in low doses but be uricosuric (increase elimination) in high doses. An example is aspirin. The extent of the effect is modified by the acidity of the urine.

Almost all diuretics, such as the thiazide diuretics used to treat hypertension (see above), except spironolactone, will tend to cause hyperuricaemia by reducing renal elimination of urate.

Other diseases

Insulin-dependent diabetes is not usually associated with hyperuricaemia, except when diabetic control is extremely poor and body fats are metabolised, resulting in diabetic ketosis. These ketones will cause a transient severe hyperuricaemia by reducing renal excretion of urate. However, with correction of the ketosis, the hyperuricaemia will revert to normal. The main problem is the associated insulin resistance in the diabetic which, if sustained and associated with obesity, may promote both hypertriglyceridaemia and hyperuricaemia.

Untreated hypothyroidism (reduced thyroid function) is often associated with hyperuricaemia, as are disorders of the parathyroid glands. In each case, restoration of normal hormonal function or replacement hormone therapy will correct the hyperuricaemia.

Hyperuricaemia is found in a wide range of acute medical conditions. Increased turnover of the bone marrow, such as occurs in marrow malignancies, leukaemias, marrow proliferative disorders and infectious mononucleosis (glandular fever), can lead to an increase in urate production. Greater body acidity in the form of a respiratory acidosis or inadequate oxygenation of tissues, as occurs in respiratory failure, can again promote hyperuricaemia. Psoriasis, by increasing the turnover of skin cells, can also cause hyperuricaemia.

All of these generalised diseases cause hyperuricaemia by an effect on either purine degradation and/or urate production or on the elimination of urate by the kidney.

Summary

- Genetic over-production is a rare but important cause of hyperuricaemia.
- Rates of urate excretion vary widely, and under-excretion can exist independently of other kidney problems.
- Kidney disease can cause under-excretion; if the kidney disease can be treated the excretion rate can improve.
- High body weight is closely associated with high serum urate concentration and a reduction in body weight with a reduction in urate concentration.
- Although the purine content of the diet contributes to the urate load, a diet that complies with Heart Foundation recommendations is unlikely to cause problems for most gout sufferers.
- High alcohol consumption increases urate production through increased breakdown of ATP, and decreases urate excretion.
- High blood fat (triglycerides) found with hyperuricaemia may be an early warning of cardiovascular disease.
- Diuretics prescribed for high blood pressure lead to the development of hyperuricaemia.
- Some other medications and acute diseases can contribute to hyperuricaemia.

six

Urate crystal formation

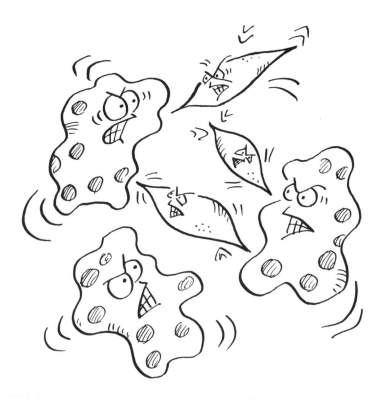

Why and how do urate crystals form within the body?
What effect do they have?

Acute gout is a response by inflammatory cells to the formation of urate crystals. Thus, there are two components to consider in an acute attack of gout: the factors that cause the crystals to be formed, and why and how cells react to the formation of these crystals.

Urate solubility: why do urate crystals form?

As with the crystallisation of any salt from a solution, urate crystallises when its solubility in the solution is exceeded; that is, when there is more urate present than can stay dissolved. However, the situation in serum in the body is not as simple as in water in a test-tube because there are many other substances also dissolved in the serum which can affect the solubility. Of these, some factors preferentially maintain urate in solution and others promote its conversion to crystals.

Some of these include:

- the concentration of urate
- pH (acidity or alkalinity)
- temperature
- solubilising proteins, and
- local factors.

The concentration of urate

The concentration of urate at the site of crystal formation is ultimately the most important determining factor. If the concentration of the urate exceeds its solubility under the conditions applying at any site, then a crystal will form, and this may act as a seed for other crystals to be formed.

There are two special situations to consider. The first is in a joint (such as the big toe joint) where the local concentration of urate might also depend on the passage of water from within the joint fluid to outside the joint, thereby increasing the concentration of all substances within the joint fluid, including urate. Thus, the ability of urate to pass through the lining membrane of the joint in comparison with the ability of water to pass through that membrane might be important. The second special situation applies to the kidney, which concentrates the substances it is eliminating from the body. The concentration of uric acid in the urine is always many times that of urate in other tissues and, depending on other factors, this may constitute a risk of forming uric acid crystals within the kidney tubules.

pH

The pH (acidity or alkalinity) of the dissolving fluid affects the solubility of urate, since the higher the pH (the more alkaline the fluid) the more soluble the urate becomes, and the lower the pH (more acid) the less soluble urate becomes. This is not as important as it might seem since the body pH is tightly controlled (buffered) to minimise major deviations of blood and tissue pH from the normal of 7.4. However, the kidney excretes hydrogen ions from the body, and these make the urine persistently acid. There can be a wide variation in pH within the tubular fluid and in the urine, and therefore a widely varying risk of urate or uric acid crystal or stone formation. However, the factors involved in the kidney are different from those in the tissues, and each needs to be looked upon as a special case.

Temperature

Just as cooling promotes crystal formation in a test-tube solution, cooling of tissues can promote crystal formation. The human body tends to maintain an even body temperature at about 37 °C and the flow of blood to tissues tends to maintain this. However, the body extremities and the peripheral joints may become colder under certain circumstances, and such cooling may enable urate crystals to form in the fingers and toes.

Solubilising proteins

Solubilising proteins are important in keeping urate in solution. Whereas urate in a watery or salt solution may crystallise out at a concentration above, say, 0.5 mmol/L, urate may stay dissolved in blood plasma at a concentration exceeding 1 or 2 mmol/L, that is twice to four times as much stays dissolved. This is believed to be because certain proteins in the blood plasma maintain urate in soluble form at these much higher concentrations.

Local factors

A variety of local tissue constituents act to keep urate in solution in tissues. If these tissue factors are broken down, the ability to maintain urate in solution may be lost and urate may be crystallised in the tissues. This might account for the tendency of urate to deposit in certain tissues such as cartilage.

Other factors

A variety of other factors may also precipitate acute gout by mechanisms which we understand only poorly. These include an injury or operation, a major alteration in urate concentration (such as happens when urate-lowering treatment is stopped) or indiscreet use of alcohol. Many other factors may cause an acute attack of gout to develop out of the blue, but we do not understand why. What we do know is that those factors which cause fluctuation in the urate concentration in the blood and in the tissues can often precipitate an acute attack of gout.

Despite being able to list many precipitating factors, in many cases we still do not understand why urate comes out of solution and forms crystals. As already indicated, the risk of developing a sudden attack of gout at a serum urate concentration of 0.54 mmol/L is only one in 20, so that only one out of 20 patients with this particular serum urate concentration is likely to develop gout in any one year. However, of 20 such patients, we cannot identify which patient with a serum urate of this level is the one most likely to develop an attack of gout in that particular year.

What are urate crystals like?

When urate crystals form in the body, they are usually in the form of monosodium urate monohydrate (MSUM). These crystals are about the size of a white blood cell and range from 5 to 25 microns in length. They are often called acicular, which means that they are shaped like a needle.

Certain characteristics of the crystals enable them to be identified readily under the microscope. The first is that they are brilliantly refractile (reflective) when viewed under polarised light, so that urate crystals can be identified in any joint fluid by examining the fluid for these minute crystals under polarised light. A special microscope with a rotating stage and an attachment called a red plate compensator can be used to identify them even more clearly. Seen through this device, MSUM (or urate) crystals are very different from all other crystals forming within the body. (In technical terms, they are birefringent crystals, yellow in the line of slow vibration of light through the red plate compensator.)

The situation is different in the kidney where the urate is more concentrated and subjected to a low pH. At this low pH (high acidity), more of the urate is in the form of uric acid and this becomes less soluble as the acidity of the urine increases (or the pH falls). In this situation, the uric acid crystals are shapeless (amorphous) and do not form the characteristic needle shape. In addition, high urinary uric acid excretions are associated with two different types of uric acid stones or calculi, the first being a uric acid calculus (which does not show on an X-ray) and the other being a calcium oxalate calculus (which does show as an opaque mass on an X-ray). However, these develop not within the collecting ducts of the tubules but rather within the kidney pelvis (the part adjoining the ureter) and the ureter itself.

How do different tissues and cells respond?

In most parts of the body, body cells respond to the formation of urate crystals in much the same way as they respond to the presence of other foreign material (such as bacteria) within the tissues.

The common cell involved with this response is the polymorphonuclear leucocyte, often referred to as a polymorph or white blood cell (*poly* many, *morpho* shape, therefore white cell with many nucleus shapes). These cells respond to crystal formation by releasing a variety of chemical messengers or factors which attract other polymorph cells, thereby increasing the response. They also release a range of inflammatory mediators which are intended to improve the ability of the body to respond to the foreign body and to eliminate or isolate it if possible. In the process, the polymorphs may engulf the crystal and some may partially digest it (figure 2.2).

It is this polymorph response to the crystals which causes the inflammation of acute gout and which often makes it difficult to distinguish between an acute joint inflammation (or arthritis) caused by crystals and that caused by bacteria. It is this response, too, which is inhibited by the drug colchicine when it is used as a preventative (prophylactic) against acute attacks of gout.

Other tissue cells and cells lining either the joint cavity or the bursae may respond to crystal formation in a less dramatic way. For example, the cells lining the renal tubules may ingest urate and uric acid crystals when they come in contact with them. This response may be determined by physical and chemical similarities between the cell surface membrane and the crystals.

Whereas some crystal-induced diseases seem to occur from the rupture of a deposit of pre-formed crystals, in gout it seems that urate crystals are formed within joint fluid and stay as single crystals until they provoke a cellular response.

What switches off the acute attack of gout?

Acute gout will often settle down within two weeks, even without treatment. Crystals are still present as the acute gout subsides, but something makes the inflammatory cells less responsive to them.

The protein coating which forms on the crystal is important in determining the vigour of the cellular response. Thus, a coating of a substance called immunoglobulin G makes the crystal much more likely to excite a response by polymorphs, whereas a coating of apolipoprotein E has the reverse effect. A variety of proteoglycans (components of cartilage) coating the crystals also protect against the induction of a cellular response. We need to know a lot more about what makes some crystals produce an inflammatory cellular response while

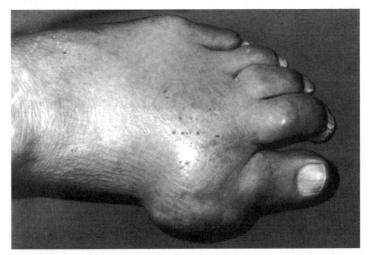

Figure 6.1 A large tophus affecting the bunion joint following years of inadequate treatment.

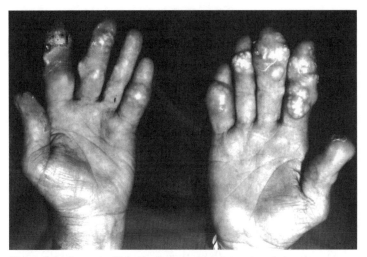

Figure 6.2 Large tophi on the fingers which have ulcerated and discharged. This patient's hyperuricaemia had never been treated and he had suffered recurrent attacks of gout for more than twenty years.

others have no effect. This is particularly important because the deposition of crystals as tophi is not usually associated with any response by inflammatory cells.

Urate crystal deposits responsible for an acute attack of gout are usually visible only under a microscope. However, in a tophus this crystal deposit becomes so massive that it can be seen with the naked eye (figure 6.1). Tophi are most readily seen just beneath the skin.

In the days before treatment was available for the hyperuricaemia which caused them, they could become bigger than a hen's egg, and might discharge their white chalky contents (figure 6.2). This white chalky material is said to have been used at one time by a teacher for writing on a blackboard! Such accounts emphasise how gross gout was in previous centuries and how rarely such severe manifestations are seen in the twentieth century.

Tophi may resorb or dissolve away completely if treatment for the gout brings the concentration of urate in the surrounding tissue fluid low enough (usually less than 0.30 mmol/L).

X-rays and gout

An X-ray of a joint which has been the subject of a single acute attack of gout rarely shows anything abnormal. In the acute attack, the soft tissues around a joint may increase in size and thickness and, although soft tissues cannot often be seen clearly on X-rays, this may show. Thus, any asymmetry in a joint, due both to the local inflammation and any microscopic deposits of urate, may indicate that it has been involved in inflammation.

Urate crystals or deposits do not themselves show on X-rays, i.e. they are radiolucent (X-rays pass through without being absorbed). All one can see is their effect. If these crystals are deposited in bone, they may replace a portion of bone. Because X-rays can pass through them they appear as a hole in the solid or opaque bone. Thus, urate deposits around joints affected by gout may appear as punched-out areas within the bone or they may appear as radiolucent areas with overhanging margins near the joint surface (figure 6.3). These holes are patchy and asymmetrical. Most importantly, they do not develop early in gout. These radiological or X-ray changes of gout may strongly suggest and be consistent with a diagnosis of gout but are rarely enough on their own for a diagnosis to be made.

Usually, a patient has suffered from gout for 5–10 years before consistent changes develop in bone and show up on an X-ray. Thus, the radiological changes in gout are characteristically late in appearing and usually show up only in a joint that has been affected by many attacks of gout. Such gouty changes will be seen more frequently in peripheral joints than in central joints, more commonly in the feet than in the hands, and more commonly in the toes than in the fingers. Involvement of the spine and trunk joints is much less common.

When hyperuricaemia is corrected and urate concentrations are restored to normal, urate deposits or tophi are gradually resorbed, although large tophi may take many years to disappear. Thus, the radiological changes may heal over time.

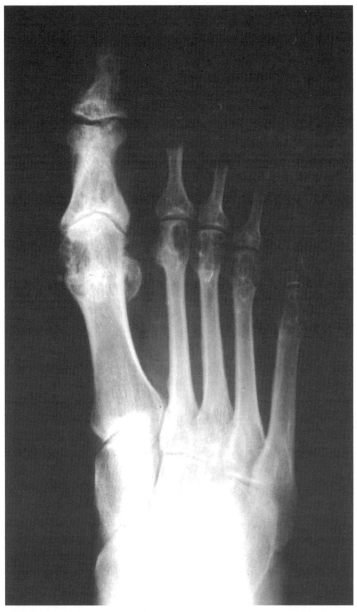

Figure 6.3 X-ray of a gouty foot.

Summary

- Urate crystals form when the urate concentration exceeds the amount that can stay dissolved at the temperature and acidity of the joint fluids.
- The extremities tend to be cooler than the rest of the body, so crystal formation is more common in the fingers and toes.
- Urate crystals are easily identified with a microscope using polarised light.
- The body initially responds to the crystals in the same way as it responds to invading bacteria. This response gradually subsides.
- Gout usually needs to have been present for many years before it produces changes that show up on X-ray.

seven

Gout and the kidney

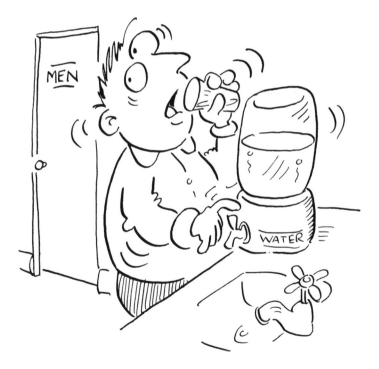

What does the kidney do?

How does it do it?

How does this relate to gout?

The normal kidney

When a person is found to have both gout and kidney disease, one must consider whether the kidney disease could be due to (secondary to) the gout, or whether the gout could be secondary to the kidney disease.

We need to begin with how the kidney normally functions in relation to uric acid or urate.

The main kidney structures are shown in figure 7.1.

The kidney is very important in determining the urate concentration in the blood and tissue fluid because it excretes two-thirds of the urate which is produced each day and must be eliminated. (The remainder passes into the small bowel in the intestinal secretions.)

As shown in figure 3.2, blood is first filtered at a glomerulus (a minute filtering sphere) and then the filtrate passes along fine tubules from which constituents desirable for the body can be reabsorbed and retained, and undesirable constituents can be excreted. Most of this reabsorption and secretion takes place in the convoluted (twisting) tubule. Most of the concentration of the undesirable bodily constituents to be eliminated in urine occurs in a loop of the tubules which goes down into the depth of the kidney near the kidney pelvis, the so-called renal medulla. In this way, the protein-free blood filtrate is concentrated in the tubule, where its composition is modified so as to pass into the tubular fluid those components which the body needs to eliminate. Several filtering units may pass into the one common collecting duct and many such collecting ducts may then flow into the renal pelvis, which is the common collecting system for the whole kidney. From the renal pelvis, a small tube (the ureter), about 2 mm in internal diameter, passes down from the kidney to the bladder. When the bladder empties, the urine passes out from the body through the urethra.

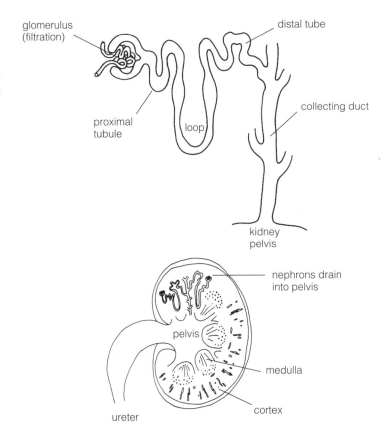

Figure 7.1 The kidney unit (nephron) and its various components.

The amount of urate which passes from the blood filtrate into the kidney pelvis is about 10 per cent of the amount which is filtered. Various factors influence the amount of urate which is reabsorbed or secreted from the kidney and ultimately control the amount of urate excreted. Important among these are the amount of water and salt and the amount of hydrogen ion (acid) eliminated in the urine. The elimination of hydrogen ions in the urine by the kidney is what makes the urine acidic, and it needs to be remembered that uric acid is less soluble in an acidic solution.

Kidney damage due to gout

As in other parts of the body, the adverse effects of gout arise as a result of the formation of crystals of urate and uric acid. The kidney is particularly susceptible to such problems because so much urate passes through the kidney in its elimination from the body and because a major function of the kidney is to concentrate the fluid passing through it.

As discussed in chapter 6, three important factors in urate crystallisation are the concentration of urate, the pH or acidity of the fluid, and the presence or absence of solubilising factors that maintain urate in solution. The normal function of the kidney increases the first two of these factors that promote crystal formation: the kidney acts to concentrate most constituents of the fluid passing through it, including urate, and it increases its acidity as the tubular fluid passes from the cortex of the kidney down toward the medulla and into the kidney pelvis.

When, in previous centuries, gout was severe and untreatable, repeated attacks of gout would lead to the formation of tophi, and some of these tophi would form within the kidney. The cellular response at the sites of crystal formation could lead to kidney disease, causing high blood pressure (hypertension). The hypertension resulting from tophi forming within a kidney could then aggravate the tendency to vascular disease, which could go on to cause further kidney disease. Thus, in the untreated state, the development of tophi in the kidney could lead to hypertension, and both the tophi and the hypertension could aggravate the underlying kidney disease or kidney failure. In general, the risk of developing this type of kidney disease was proportional to the severity or the degree of hyperuricaemia. Thus, in times past, many patients with severe tophaceous gout would develop kidney disease and could proceed to develop kidney failure with vascular disease, with all the potential complications that affect the heart and blood vessels.

That was before effective treatments became available. Today, many patients with gout still worry that their gout will progress to cause kidney disease, so it cannot be emphasised too much that if gout is treated effectively, and the serum urate is restored to normal, the risk of formation of tophi within the kidney becomes negligible. If the serum urate in a gouty patient is normal, that patient is at no greater risk of kidney disease than a person without gout. Kidney disease of this type is currently seen only in patients with tophaceous gout who, for one reason or another, do not achieve a normal serum urate concentration.

Our studies of patients with both gout and kidney disease suggest that kidney disease does not develop in patients with primary gout until patients have had an average of 20 attacks of gout over a period of 5–10 years. However, as will be discussed in the next chapter, the patient with gout may have other risk factors for cardiovascular disease, and these may persist even when the serum urate is normal and may, in themselves, contribute to the development of kidney disease on a vascular, or blood vessel, basis.

High urine uric acid

The distinction has already been drawn between the concentration of uric acid or urate in the blood plasma and tissue fluid and that in the urine. A high concentration of uric acid in urine can occur without the presence of gout or even, in the early stages, without the presence of hyperuricaemia. Accordingly, a high concentration of uric acid in urine is in itself a risk factor for the development of kidney disease, separate from a high urate concentration in the blood.

There are four main situations when a high urine uric acid will occur and may cause kidney damage:

- genetic overproduction or inherited over-excretion of urate
- increased breakdown of cell nuclei
- uricosuric therapy, and
- high dietary purine consumption.

Genetic overproduction or inherited over-excretion of urate

Genetic over-production of urate has already been referred to as occurring in HPRT deficiency (page 44). It can also occur in rare inherited disorders of the kidney tubules where urate cannot be reabsorbed and where there is a very high urine urate.

These situations are rare and would not be seen in 99 per cent of gout sufferers. However, the study of rare conditions such as these can aid understanding of the more common disease mechanisms.

Increased breakdown of cell nuclei

Increased breakdown of cell nuclei is most commonly seen following chemotherapy for cancers. Chemotherapy acts by destroying the cancerous cells and, when the nuclei of these cells are degraded, it results in a great increase in the production of urate. This large urate load needs to be disposed of, and the greatest part of it is eliminated by the kidney. The load may be so great that some of the kidney tubules are blocked by uric acid crystal deposits, preventing their particular nephrons from functioning. This problem is now usually anticipated during chemotherapy and is prevented by judicious use of the drug allopurinol (to suppress the urate production) and maintenance of a large volume of alkaline urine (to increase the solubility of the urate and reduce crystal formation).

Uricosuric therapy

Uricosuric drug treatment lowers the serum urate by increasing the urine uric acid excretion. This therapy will be discussed in more detail in chapter 12.

The increased urinary uric acid excretion may be a problem if the uric acid concentration and pH of the urine are such as will allow uric acid crystals to form within the tubule or collecting duct. Usually preventative strategies are put in place, but the potential for crystal formation may still persist. The increase in urinary uric acid is only mild when the patient is stabilised on the uricosuric drug, but the risk of crystal formation from a high urinary uric acid may recur if therapy is stopped and re-started.

High dietary purine consumption

A large intake of purines or increased urate production such as can occur after heavy alcohol consumption can lead to a sudden load of urate being presented to the kidneys for elimination. This creates the same potential for uric acid crystals to form within the renal tubule as high urate concentrations from any other cause.

Kidney damage from high urinary uric acid

As already mentioned, amorphous (shapeless) crystals of uric acid can form within the renal tubules or within the renal pelvis if the concentration of uric acid and the pH of the fluid is appropriate. It should be stressed again that these crystals are different from the urate crystals (MSUM) which occur in interstitial tissues and joint or tissue fluid. If diagnosed and treated early, these uric acid crystals can be washed out of the tubule and renal function restored to normal. This is achieved by altering both the concentration and pH of the tubular fluid, i.e. by alkalinising the fluid and by producing a large flow rate of dilute urine. The potential for reversing this type of kidney damage needs to be remembered if there is any sudden deterioration of renal function in a patient with a high urine uric acid.

The damage from blockage of a tubule tends to occur mainly within the collecting ducts, although occasionally it can occur in the renal pelvis or ureter. In either of these latter positions, the crystals may clump together to produce renal calculi or renal stones. In many cases these stones consist not of uric acid but of calcium oxalate. Thus, both uric acid as well as calcium oxalate calculi in the renal pelvis may be a hazard of a sustained high urinary uric acid concentration from any cause.

The risk factors for forming calcium oxalate calculi are not all understood, but the absence of certain solubilising factors seems to be important. However, the presence of other aggravating factors such as a high urinary uric acid concentration is also important. Uric acid calculi cannot be seen on X-rays, whereas calcium oxalate calculi are radio-opaque and can be seen on plain X-rays.

Thus, while crystals may block the tubules, calculi or stones may form within the renal pelvis, ureter or bladder, where they can cause their own problems of infection, obstruction, bleeding or pain. In each case, the risk of forming calculi is greatly reduced by the maintenance of a dilute, alkaline urine or by the administration of allopurinol.

The presence of uric acid crystals within a renal tubule has two effects. First, it may block the flow of tubular fluid along that tubule and this may stop the functioning of the renal unit or nephron. Second, the tubular lining cells may interact with the crystals, ingesting them and digesting and degrading them. If this is incomplete the crystals may pass beneath the tubular lining cells and through the tubular basement membrane, where they may become a focus for the formation of urate (MSUM) crystals within the tissue between the renal tubules, resulting in the formation of renal microtophi.

It is better to prevent the formation of uric acid crystals. The maintenance of a dilute urine is desirable for any patient with a uric acid problem. However, if this is insufficient, the administration of allopurinol will greatly reduce the risk of complications from a high urinary uric acid. It should be stressed that renal tubular damage from uric acid crystal obstruction may be reversible and the tubular cells may recover after appropriate treatment.

Gout secondary to primary renal disease

The situation is completely different when a patient has kidney disease first and then develops gout because of the kidney disease.

In this situation, the hyperuricaemia is caused by the reduced ability of the kidney to eliminate urate due to the associated loss of glomeruli or functioning filtration units. Gout is not a problem with most varieties of chronic renal disease, and gout secondary to primary renal disease occurs in less than 5 per cent of such patients. The risk of developing gout relates to the severity of the hyperuricaemia, and in many varieties of chronic renal disease compensatory mechanisms prevent excessive hyperuricaemia (usually by increased elimination into the small bowel) so that disproportionate hyperuricaemia does not occur. Unless the hyperuricaemia is unusually severe, a moderate degree of hyperuricaemia will usually have been present in patients with primary renal disease for at least 10 years before the patient develops any gout.

The tendency to develop hyperuricaemia will be aggravated by the presence of other factors which might cause elevation of the serum urate, such as the co-administration of diuretic tablets.

Four varieties of primary renal disease have been recognised as being associated with a higher incidence of gout:

- inherited primary renal disease
- kidney damage resulting from lead poisoning
- polycystic disease of the kidneys, and
- analgesic-induced kidney disease.

Inherited primary renal disease

Several varieties of inherited primary renal disease, often resulting in small shrunken kidneys, are associated with disproportionate hyperuricaemia and the later development of gout. Medullary cystic disease is one such inherited kidney disease.

Kidney damage resulting from lead poisoning

A form of kidney damage called chronic lead nephropathy may occur after lead poisoning or the long-term ingestion of lead in childhood or a more serious degree of chronic lead poisoning in adults. This is associated with disproportionate hyper-uricaemia and a 50 per cent incidence of gout.

Polycystic disease of the kidneys

Polycystic disease of the kidneys has been associated with gout in many patients, although recent studies have placed doubt on this finding. The precise mechanism by which polycystic kidney disease could contribute to gout is not well understood.

Analgesic-induced kidney disease

There is a small body of evidence to suggest that analgesic-induced kidney disease (caused by excessive consumption of APC-aspirin, phenacetin and caffeine), with damage especially involving the kidney tubules, may induce under-excretion of urate and so have an association with the development of gout.

Clinical patterns of gout and kidney disease

In some patients with both gout and kidney disease the gout came first and the kidney disease came second, and in others the kidney disease came first and the gout came second. In the absence of clear evidence from the medical record or from the patient's history as to which came first, one can only see how well the patient fits in with the characteristic clinical pattern of one or the other group.

In the gout-first group, patients tend to be older, the gout is usually more frequent and severe, more joints tend to be involved and the gout is more frequently tophaceous. In this group, renal disease is usually seen only after 10 years and at least 20 attacks of gout.

In the group in whom the renal disease occurred first, characteristically the patients are younger, the gout is less frequent and severe, fewer joints are involved, tophi are infrequent, and usually renal disease had been present for about 10 years before the development of the gout.

Renal stones (calculi) and gout

Sufferers from gout have problems because uric acid crystallises within their joints. They may also have problems with uric acid crystallising in the urinary tract because this is the major route for uric acid elimination from the body. In fact, before their first attack of gouty arthritis at least 10 per cent of gout sufferers have had an episode of renal colic due to the formation of a small stone (calculus) within the kidney or the urinary tract. These calculi, which may vary in size from a millimetre to several centimetres, commonly cause intense pain (renal colic) which passes around the loin to the groin on the same side; this may be accompanied by the passage of blood in the urine (haematuria). Often the stones are small enough to be passed out of the body in the urine without any problem, but occasionally they may be large enough to cause obstruction to urine flow, and this may be complicated by infection in the urinary tract.

Many of these stones are made of uric acid and therefore do not show up in a plain X-ray of the abdomen. In patients with uric acid stones, the concentration of uric acid in the urine is usually normal, but the urine is much more acid than usual, and this is what makes the uric acid crystallise out. (The urine of these patients may be one hundred or more times more acid than the blood.) The exact cause of this high urinary acidity in many gout patients is not well understood. It is found in many people with gout in the absence of any other signs of kidney disease.

The other type of kidney stone common in patients with gout is a calcium oxalate stone. This is usually associated with a very high urinary uric acid excretion, but the urine need not be unusually acid. Often this high urinary uric acid seems to be caused by a diet high in purines. The reasons why a high urinary uric acid should promote the formation of another type of calculus are complex and involve solubilising factors in the urine which would normally maintain the calcium oxalate in solution. Since the stones contain calcium, which is opaque to X-rays, calcium oxalate calculi can usually be detected by a plain X-ray of the abdomen.

Another very important factor promoting calculus formation is a poor urine volume (less than 1400 mL per 24 hours). This is something which all gout patients need to bear in mind because they can readily increase their urine volume by increasing their water consumption.

How can renal stones be prevented?

The first thing that a gout sufferer can do to reduce the risk of stones forming within the urinary tract is to maintain a dilute urine, i.e. always drink sufficient fluid to have a urine volume exceeding 1500 mL/day. Few other manoeuvres have as great an effect upon the uric acid concentration in the urine as the volume of urine passed or the urine flow rate.

If you have had a renal stone in the past, the urine volume should be kept even higher, at 2 litres per 24 hours or more. This will usually require a fluid intake of at least 3 litres per 24 hours.

Because both uric acid and calcium oxalate calculi are associated with relatively high uric acid concentrations in the urine, the risk of calculi can be reduced by the administration of allopurinol. This drug, which will be discussed in more detail later, reduces the amount of uric acid in all body fluids (including the urine) so that the amount of uric acid excreted and its concentration is less.

In patients known to have a high urine uric acid, it may be wise to avoid using drugs which will increase the concentration of uric acid in the urine, such as the uricosuric drugs. However,

GOUT AND THE KIDNEY

sometimes, as in a patient sensitive to allopurinol, it may not be possible to avoid their use. In these cases it is vital that the patient maintain a high urine volume and that the urine be kept neutral or mildly alkaline, i.e. approximate pH of 7. However, the most important way a gout patient can help prevent or treat a renal calculus is to get into a habit of drinking plenty of water and thereby maintaining a good urine flow rate.

Summary

- The kidney filters urate from the blood, but much of this is later reabsorbed and only about 10 per cent is excreted.
- Uric acid can crystallise out in the kidney or urinary tract if the urine is concentrated and very acid.
- Uric acid crystals can damage the kidney, but the damage can often be prevented and reversed by maintaining a dilute alkaline urine.
- There are two types of kidney stone associated with gout. Calcium oxalate stones will show on an X-ray but uric acid stones do not.
- Kidney disease leading to reduced excretion of urate can result in gout.

eight

Gout and the blood vessels

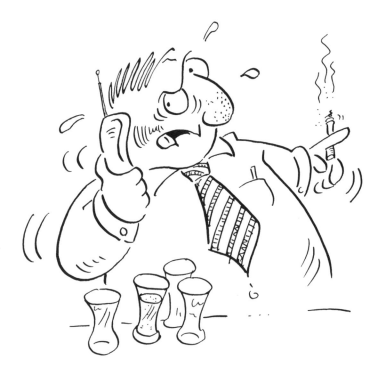

Can gout cause cardiovascular disease?

In the centuries before gout became treatable, patients with gout suffered an increased risk of vascular (blood vessel) disease, and up to half died of stroke or heart disease. As a result, gout was associated with a shortened life span. In fact, Huchard was recorded in the last century as saying 'Gout is to the arteries what rheumatism (rheumatic fever) is to the heart,' in other words, just as an attack of rheumatic fever frequently led to damage to the heart valves, the development of gout frequently led to disease of the arteries.

Since disease of the blood vessels still poses the biggest risk of severe disability or premature death in the community, we need to examine whether Huchard's statement still holds true now that effective treatment can correct the hyperuricaemia of gout.

How are blood vessels affected by disease?

The healthy functioning of all the major organs in the body depends upon a good supply of blood and this may be interfered with by disease of the arteries restricting the blood supply. Disease of arteries is common, often from a surprisingly young age, and causes its greatest problems when it affects the blood vessels which supply the vital organs such as the heart, the brain and the kidneys, and the blood vessels to the limbs, particularly the legs.

Disease affecting the arteries is referred to as either arteriosclerosis (sclerosis meaning hardening of the arteries) or atherosclerosis (atheroma referring to the fatty streaks that often underlie the plaques which develop in the artery walls). Its formation is patchy and unpredictable. If there is sufficient disease of the artery wall to reduce the blood flow in an artery to a vital organ or structure such as the brain, major problems can arise with the function of the affected organ. When reduced blood flow affects the heart, it is referred to as a heart attack or a coronary occlusion (blockage of the coronary artery which supplies the heart muscle). If it affects the brain, reduced blood flow can produce either a major or a minor stroke, depending on the degree of blockage and the blood vessel and particular areas of the brain involved. The healthy functioning of the kidney likewise depends on sufficient blood flow, and disease of the blood vessels to the kidney can interfere with kidney function and can also cause hypertension (high blood pressure). Finally, disease of the arteries supplying the limbs, particularly the lower limbs, can lead to poor circulation and inadequate peripheral blood supply.

Several factors are known to increase the risk of developing vascular disease. The most common are an elevated serum cholesterol (hypercholesterolaemia) and a raised blood pressure (hypertension), both of which are aggravated by the third factor of overweight or obesity. The fourth important factor is cigarette smoking. Other factors promoting atherosclerosis or degenerative vascular disease include inherited factors (which are not well understood) and factors which promote the formation of clots within the vascular system, particularly the deposition of platelets on the surface of atherosclerotic plaques at critical positions in blood vessels. Elevation of blood fats (triglycerides) may also contribute, but triglycerides are less important than cholesterol.

The long-standing concern that the development of gout would lead to or aggravate atherosclerosis is reinforced by the finding that many patients with coronary artery disease have elevated uric acid concentrations and, in some, this leads to the development of gout. However, evidence of an association between gout and atherosclerosis does not mean that gout has necessarily caused the atherosclerosis or even that the atherosclerosis has caused the gout. It is important to note that, along with the development of effective treatment for gout, there has been a significant reduction in the incidence of vascular disease in the community over the last 20–30 years, in both nongouty and gouty patients.

Hyperuricaemia and vascular disease

Where does the patient with gout stand with the problem of associated vascular disease? Does the presence of a high uric acid concentration of itself increase the risk of vascular disease and, if so, by what mechanism?

It is clear that many patients with gout have a number of conditions associated with their hyperuricaemia which may independently increase the risk of vascular disease. Thus, one type of gout, seen in over half the patients today, is associated with overweight (obesity), with regular alcohol consumption, with high blood triglyceride (fat) levels, and often with hypertension. Each of these factors can independently cause hyperuricaemia. In addition, both being overweight and taking alcohol regularly can increase the serum triglyceride concentration, and the abnormal blood lipids (fats) increase the degree of atherosclerosis or degenerative vascular disease (figure 5.1). In this situation, the basic problem is the obesity which leads to both the elevated blood lipids and the hyperuricaemia. However, although associated, the hyperuricaemia is not the cause of the raised triglycerides and the degenerative vascular disease. Looked at in this way, the hyperuricaemia is an 'innocent bystander' to the development of vascular disease, with the factors which cause the vascular disease also contributing to the hyperuricaemia. This means that correcting the hyperuricaemia by drugs directed at lowering urate concentrations would have no effect on the vascular disease.

One theory suggests that the hyperuricaemia is directly responsible for an increase in platelet adhesiveness or stickiness. This increased stickiness would result in the development of deposits of blood platelets on the walls of the blood vessels which may cause localised narrowing. There have been many studies to try to demonstrate or define a predictable effect of a high urate concentration in the blood on platelet adhesiveness or stickiness. These studies have been technically difficult both to carry out and to interpret. The general consensus is that none has shown consistent changes and that there is not much evidence that the degree of hyperuricaemia seen in our gouty patients has any direct adverse effect on the blood vessels.

However, even if hyperuricaemia is an innocent bystander to the process of the development of vascular disease, this does not mean that, having treated the hyperuricaemia, one should ignore any associated vascular disease or the vascular risk. Any vascular risk factors promoting atherosclerosis in a patient with gout need to be tackled in their own right and their correction will often benefit the hyperuricaemia. Thus excessive body weight, excessive or regular alcohol consumption, hyperlipidaemia, hypertension, impaired glucose tolerance and cigarette smoking all need to be controlled in a patient with gout. Sometimes, the gout is the outward and visible signal that all is not well with a patient's general health. Thus, an attack of gout must not be viewed in isolation from the rest of a patient's health.

Longevity and gout

Life insurance policies once penalised patients with gout in the belief that they had an increased mortality (particularly from vascular disease) and shorter life expectancy, but it is now thought that there is no significant increase in mortality associated with gout and there is no longer any need for the loading of life insurance policies. An attack of gout in itself need have no real significance in so far as longevity is concerned. It should be stressed again, however, how important it is to look for other risk factors for vascular disease in a patient with gout and to treat these on their own merits. If these can be controlled or corrected, the patient's life expectancy should be completely normal.

Summary

- Historically, gout patients frequently suffered kidney damage that led to hypertension and cardiovascular problems.
- Gout patients often also have high blood fats, which is a risk factor for cardiovascular disease.

- Obesity, high alcohol consumption and hypertension contribute to both hyperuricaemia and cardiovascular disease.
- Although gout does not cause cardiovascular disease, controlling the risk factors for one can often improve the other.
- Any vascular risk factors need to be treated regardless of any lack of association with gout.

nine

How to manage your gout

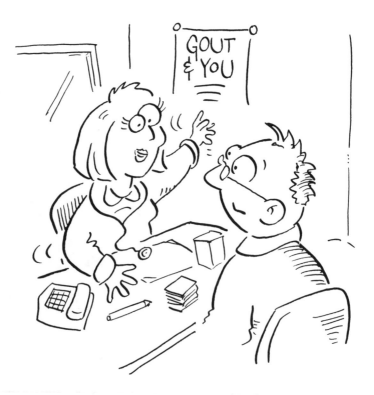

When should an acute attack be treated?
How can attacks be prevented?

Many aspects of the management of gout require close collaboration between yourself as the patient and your medical
adviser. You need to understand how, why and when to treat
your gout, and your doctor needs to know which are the best
drugs to give you and when is the appropriate time. In a
chronic (long-standing) disease such as gout, there is rarely a
permanent cure. Rather, it is a condition which can be controlled, and a satisfactory relationship between you and your
doctor is vital for success. As part of this partnership, you need
to be as informed as possible about your condition.

The advice I will give you is a consensus overview of the best
ways to manage gout. However, the management plan needs
to be adapted to the needs of each particular individual.
Accordingly, any advice I will give needs to be adapted to your
particular needs and circumstances. In particular, all medications have the potential to cause side-effects and these vary
from patient to patient; the risk of particular side-effects may
dominate the choice of a particular drug therapy. Therefore,
although the general advice I will give should apply in the great
majority of patients, there will be many occasions when your
doctor needs to approach your problem differently.

How to manage acute attacks of gout

Details of drug treatment will be included in the next chapter,
but certain principles are essential for successful management.

Ensure correct diagnosis

Correct diagnosis of gout is absolutely essential for effective
management. If everything about your gout is completely typical, there may be no doubt about the diagnosis and, corre-
spondingly, appropriate treatment can be chosen. If, however,
there is anything atypical or unusual about the symptoms and
signs, the only way of confirming the diagnosis with absolute

certainty is for the doctor to aspirate (take a sample of) some fluid from an affected joint and look for the characteristic needle-shaped urate crystals.

Treat as early during an acute attack as possible

After one or two attacks, patients can usually feel an attack of gout coming on at a very early stage. Treatment at this stage will often stop an acute attack from developing fully. This clearly is not possible on the first occasion or if there is a need to establish the diagnosis by the demonstration of urate crystals. However, once diagnosis is certain and you have responded to drug treatment on a previous occasion, it is wise to discuss with your doctor what you should do when a further attack comes on. This may be at any time of the day or night so you need to keep the chosen medication readily available. Usually a much lower dose of medication is needed if it is taken early rather than late in the attack.

Medication

The dose of medication needs to be large enough to ensure that adequate treatment is received. Choice of the drug and its dose should be planned in advance. If colchicine is being used, a full course should be started and it should be continued either until there is relief or side-effects require termination. If the medication used is a non-steroidal anti-inflammatory drug (NSAID), the dose needed will depend upon the severity of the acute attack. If treatment is begun early, gout may settle with a dose as low as one-third of that needed if treatment is begun after severe gout has become established.

Continue treatment until the acute gout has settled

This applies particularly to the non-steroidal anti-inflammatory drugs where the dose should be slowly reduced over a period of several days after the subsidence of the acute pain and inflammation.

How can I prevent further attacks of gout?

In principle, the answer to this is simple: restore the serum urate concentration to normal and keep it there. After about a year of a normal serum urate concentration, the risk of gout will have declined sufficiently for no further attacks to have occurred or at least for attacks to have become mild and infrequent.

However, in practice fluctuations in the serum urate concentration (either up or down) can precipitate acute attacks of gout; for example, too rapid a lowering of serum urate can precipitate further acute attacks of gout. This may discourage the patient and the doctor from further attempts at correcting the underlying problem.

There are only three ways in which one can minimise this problem of recurrent gout developing while the urate concentration is being reduced:

- not giving any drugs or undertaking other activities which will alter the serum urate while there is any persisting acute gout
- attempting to ensure that any changes in the serum urate concentration occur slowly, and
- using a prophylactic dose of colchicine or NSAID to protect against acute attacks of gout.

These three strategies can usually ensure that a normal serum urate can be achieved and maintained and further attacks thereby prevented.

Thus, in order to prevent gout, there are only two approaches:

- find the cause of the hyperuricaemia and correct the cause (chapter 11), or
- if the cause cannot be found or corrected, use medications to restore the serum urate to normal (chapter 12).

However, these two approaches should be undertaken only when you have no joints actively affected by gout and when major fluctuations in the serum urate concentration can be avoided. Thus, one of the golden rules is not to attempt to correct hyperuricaemia in any person who is suffering from acute gout at the time, even if that gout seems to be mild. We know that a rapidly falling serum urate concentration can lead all too often to an acute flare-up of acute gouty arthritis.

Interim control

You still need to reduce the risk of acute gout while you are waiting for your serum urate to be corrected.

There are two drugs which can prevent acute gout, neither of which has any intrinsic effect upon the serum urate concentration. These are colchicine and the group of NSAID drugs. The dose used depends on the purpose for which they are used. When they are used prophylactically (preventatively), a low dose is used each day. When they are used to treat an acute attack, a large dose is used initially, tailing off fairly rapidly as the acute gout subsides. A prophylactic (preventive) dose of colchicine ranges between 1 and 2 tablets (each of 0.5 mg) a day. This interferes with the response of the polymorph white blood cells to any urate crystals, reducing the potential for an inflammatory response. In acute gout the dose is usually sufficient to induce diarrhoea, but the prophylactic dose should not produce any gastrointestinal side-effects such as abdominal discomfort, diarrhoea or nausea. If it does, the dose should be reduced until it produces no side-effects whatsoever. There have been rare cases of muscle pains and weakness in the lower limbs in patients with kidney insufficiency who have been taking prophylactic colchicine long-term. The value of prophylactic colchicine is sufficient to justify my continuing to advise patients to use it, even if they have some renal insufficiency, although they should be advised to stop the colchicine if they develop weakness or pain in the leg muscles.

Many of the non-steroidal anti-inflammatory agents (NSAIDs) are also useful prophylactics against acute attacks of gout. However, their side-effects (to be discussed later) are potentially more serious than those of colchicine. Colchicine is therefore the preferred prophylactic agent and it is totally effective in 80 per cent of patients and ineffective in only 5 per cent. The use of prophylactic colchicine is particularly valuable in: patients with hyperuricaemia between attacks before urate-lowering therapy has been begun or during the investigation of the causes of hyperuricaemia; during therapy to lower serum urate to within the normal range, a situation in which, as we have seen, there is an increased risk of precipitating acute gout; and in patients whose serum urate has been restored to the normal range either by lifestyle or dietary modification or by the use of drugs. In this last group of patients, the risk of gout may continue for about a year of normal urate concentrations and can be reduced by continuing prophylactic colchicine. However, after a patient has had a normal serum urate and no acute attacks of gout for 12 months, the prophylactic colchicine can be stopped.

Some patients who regularly take large doses of NSAIDs to prevent frequent recurrences of gout can develop a very severe attack of gout with the formation of large tophi without warning. This is rarely a problem with colchicine prophylaxis (prevention).

When should hyperuricaemia be corrected?

Any correction of hyperuricaemia must be life-long if it is to be worthwhile. Patients who correct their hyperuricaemia for only a period of months will develop further attacks of gout when their hyperuricaemia returns, although they will usually have a further period of some months before more acute attacks recur. The patient should understand this and must be so motivated that therapy, once started, will be continued permanently, whether the hyperuricaemia is corrected by correcting the cause or by taking medication. Usually the motivation comes from having experienced the attacks.

Each person is different in the severity and extent of gout needed to persuade them that they need continuing treatment to eradicate the gout. Some people make a permanent resolve after a single attack of gout, while others may suffer acute attacks for years before they decide that they need to correct their hyperuricaemia and hence their gout. I generally advise patients to prevent further attacks when they have had two attacks or more of acute gout in a 12 month period. Some patients do not seek preventative treatment because they do not know it exists, and others feel that the acute attacks of gout can be managed so effectively with anti-inflammatory treatment that regular treatment to prevent the attacks simply is not worth the trouble. Other patients may not be persuaded to undertake urate correcting treatment until they have developed complications in the form of hypertension, renal disease or tophi.

Decision-making is rarely simple and it needs to be remembered that there are exceptions to all rules in medicine. Sometimes patients, despite the best efforts, still develop a flare-up of acute gout during treatment to lower the serum urate. This complex situation needs close medical supervision and treatment which may involve the use of both colchicine and anti-inflammatory drugs to control any acute flare-up while normalisation of the serum urate concentration proceeds.

Summary

- Treat an acute attack of gout early, making certain of the diagnosis.
- Do not attempt to modify the serum urate concentration intentionally until the acute attack has settled completely.
- Use prophylactic colchicine in an attempt to prevent further acute attacks of gout.
- Investigate the cause of the hyperuricaemia while you are without symptoms and while you are receiving prophylactic colchicine. As a result of these investigations, decide on a plan of attack to correct the hyperuricaemia. This offers two options: either correct the cause of the hyperuricaemia by modifying your lifestyle (chapter 11) or take drugs to correct the hyperuricaemia (chapter 12).

- Correct the hyperuricaemia steadily but slowly under cover of prophylactic colchicine.
- Reduce the associated risk factors for vascular disease by correcting smoking, obesity, excess alcohol, diuretic therapy and hypertension.
- Aim to achieve a serum urate concentration consistently less than 0.36 mmol/L (6 mg per 100 mL). This serum urate needs to be checked each 1–2 months for the first 6 months and, once it has been in this normal range for 6 months, it needs to be checked three-monthly for the next 1–2 years, and intermittently thereafter as indicated by the extent of its fluctuation. If it is consistently less than 0.36 mmol/L, it needs to be checked less frequently than if it is sometimes below and sometimes above this value. A serum urate above this value is inadequate for preventing gout and is a signal to the physician to find out why the medication is ineffective. Sometimes, it is simply that the patient is forgetting to take the tablet. The presence of tophi requires a lower urate concentration to be achieved (preferably less than 0.3 mmol/L (5 mg per 100 mL).
- Above all, don't intentionally do anything to modify the serum urate concentration while you are still suffering any residual acute gout. Such modification can be taken when you are completely free from gout and are adequately covered by prophylactic colchicine.

ten

Medication used to treat an acute attack of gout

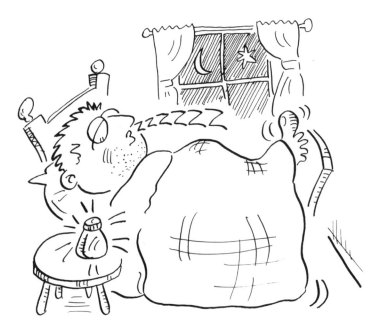

What medication is available?

What are the benefits and side-effects of each?

Only three types of medication are used to treat an acute attack of gout:

- colchicine
- corticosteroids, either by injection into the affected joint, taken orally, or by intramuscular injection, and
- non-steroidal anti-inflammatory drugs (NSAIDs).

These need to be prescribed and may need to be administered by a medical practitioner. The first couple of attacks of gout probably need to be seen by a medical practitioner, at least to establish the diagnosis. However, once the diagnosis is established, self-medication of previously prescribed medication is both necessary and desirable. The gout sufferer can usually diagnose the onset of a further acute attack accurately and at an early stage. Because early treatment can limit the duration of the attack, it is important that the person at risk of an attack of gout has access to one form of treatment which can be taken at short notice, at any hour of the day or night.

In choosing between different therapies, a physician has to weigh up both the likely success of the therapy and the risk to the individual patient of any side-effects. In regard to the attack of gout itself, its severity, the frequency of attacks and previous response to therapy will be useful guidelines. However, the seriousness and risk of side-effects varies from patient to patient, so selection of treatment needs to be individualised and there are no specific criteria which apply to all patients. The possible side-effects will be known for the individual therapies, but in each case the physician will be trying to balance the associated risks with the benefits. Thus, colchicine may be chosen if non-steroidal anti-inflammatory drugs need to be avoided. Alternatively, steroids may be administered by injection into a joint if medication cannot be taken by mouth, for example because the patient has had a recent operation, or if, for some reason, colchicine and non-steroidal anti-inflammatory drugs are not appropriate.

It is important to emphasise once again that it is vital not to do anything which will either elevate or lower the serum urate concentration while there is any persisting gouty inflammation. Thus, drugs to lower the serum urate should not be taken while there are any symptoms of gout in a joint. Likewise, drugs which are controlling the serum urate should not be stopped because an acute attack of gout has developed. If acute gout develops, it needs to be treated appropriately on its merits and, at that time, nothing should be done either to correct the associated high urate concentration or to stop drug treatment to control this. (There is only one special case when the medical practitioner may decide not to follow this rule. That is if the first administration of a drug to lower the serum urate concentration induces an acute attack of gout. In such a case, it may be desirable to stop the urate-lowering drug, but this is not a decision to be made by the patient. I accept that this advice can be a little confusing but it is a special case and does not alter the basic advice which is not to alter the serum urate during an acute attack of gout.)

Colchicine

For over 2000 years, an extract from the root of the autumn crocus, called *Colchicum autumnale*, has been used to treat gout. Since 1820, the active ingredient from this root, colchicine, has been extracted. It is available in tiny tablets containing either 0.5 or 0.6 mg of the pure substance.

Colchicine is rapidly absorbed from the stomach and intestines and distributed throughout the body, remaining in many tissues for a prolonged period. It has been shown to persist in cells as long as 10 days after the last dose was taken. The body eliminates colchicine in the bile, in the intestinal secretions and about 20 per cent in the urine. It acts by interfering with the ingestion of foreign material, such as crystals, by the polymorphonuclear leucocytes (polymorphs) which are the chief inflammatory cells in the body. It also blocks the release of factors produced by these polymorphs which call up further inflammatory cells as a response to crystal formation. It also suppresses the generation of inflammatory substances at the site of any interaction and reduces the risk of an acute attack of gout because this limits the risk of inflammation developing as a response to urate crystal formation.

The principal serious side-effects with colchicine are diarrhoea together with nausea and vomiting. The dose which produces these effects is very close to the dose needed to produce the beneficial response, and both these doses are different in every patient. Thus, the dose for treatment of an acute attack needs to be individualised. This is achieved by giving a dose of 2 tablets initially (1 mg) followed by 0.5 mg each second hour until either the acute gout subsides or the patient develops diarrhoea, vomiting or abdominal discomfort. When any of these happen, no further colchicine should be taken. Acute gout will then usually subside in 80 per cent of patients within 24 hours of development of diarrhoea. The total dose of colchicine needed may vary up to 14 tablets (7 mg) and occasionally higher than this if the patient is large. Some patients need considerably less than this and the method of administering it each 2 hours enables it to be stopped when the side-effects occur.

The amount of colchicine which each individual patient needs to treat acute gout is usually fairly constant from one attack to the next so that if a patient finds that 10 tablets (5 mg) is effective on one occasion, a dose of 9 tablets (4.5 mg) can be taken on the next occasion (again, in divided doses) and this may cause the acute attack of gout to subside without gastrointestinal side-effects.

The dose should be reduced in patients with either kidney or liver disease, in the elderly, or in those who have been receiving it on a regular basis prior to the acute attack. Overdosage is very dangerous, destroying a wide variety of cells in the body and leading to failure of many organs, and is always a life-threatening condition which may be irreversible.

No doubt it seems strange that a drug with this potential for serious side-effects is still used. However, almost all beneficial medications also have associated risks and, if used as recommended, the risk/benefit ratio of colchicine is favourable.

In some countries, colchicine is available in a preparation for intravenous use. Administration in this way does not cause any diarrhoea, vomiting, or other gastrointestinal side-effects. However, the potential for general toxicity—poisoning—is greatly increased, so there are clear recommendations for its use that must be followed. Intravenous colchicine cannot be self-administered. The drug is not available in intravenous form for use in either Australia or the United Kingdom, although it is often used in the USA.

Corticosteroids

Steroid hormones (produced naturally in the adrenal gland) and their synthetic derivatives, commonly referred to as corti-costeroids, were shown to cause a dramatic improvement in patients with the joint inflammation of rheumatoid arthritis in the 1950s. However, it was soon realised that, along with their dramatic beneficial effect, they had side-effects, many of which were almost worse than the disease for which they were given. It was also eventually appreciated that these side-effects were dose-related, increasing with larger doses. These side-effects included puffy, red changes to the face, changes of the skin leading to thinning and bruising, fluid retention and hyper-tension, an increase in the complications of peptic ulcers, development of diabetes, osteoporosis, and the flare-up of infections, including latent tuberculosis. They also inhibited the production of normal adrenal steroids by inhibiting the production of pituitary hormones and, by suppressing the patient's adrenal gland, inhibiting the response to stress. Synthetic steroids such as prednisone had similar side-effects, although, again, side-effects were dose-related.

Steroids are as effective in suppressing the inflammation of gout as they are in suppressing other inflammation. In gout, the duration of therapy is usually brief, so the side-effects are fewer. However, because early use of steroids in gout was fre-quently associated with a rebound of the acute gout after an initial subsidence, they fell into disfavour.

More recently, steroids have been reassessed in acute gout and there are reports that an appropriate selection of drug, dose and duration can prevent rebound. Thus, steroids can be used orally or by intramuscular injection in acute gout with good effect. Side-effects remain a potential problem if treatment is prolonged.

The injection of a steroid, such as methyl prednisolone, into an acutely inflamed gouty joint is a most useful form of steroid therapy, and is usually of value when a single joint is inflamed. As medical practitioners become more familiar with aspirating joints to take samples of joint fluid, this intra-articular use of steroids is becoming more frequent. However, with intra-articular injections there is the important risk that infection will be introduced into the joint, leading to the development of a septic, or infected, arthritis. Thus, intra-articular steroids should not be injected into a joint on the first attack of gout because unless some joint fluid is taken for examination it would be difficult to be sure that the problem was not septic arthritis. However, if other therapies cannot be used, intra-articular steroids may be of great value. These injections need to be administered by a medical practitioner.

Non-steroidal anti-inflammatory drugs (NSAIDs)

This name is something of a mouthful and denotes a whole group of different drugs. None has the chemical structure of a steroid, nor do they act like the adrenal steroids. Their anti-inflammatory effect is thought to occur by inhibiting a particular enzyme (prostaglandin synthetase) which allows the body cells to produce the inflammatory mediators that permit acute inflammation to occur in joints.

NSAIDs were first used to control symptoms in rheumatoid arthritis and have subsequently been used for a number of non-bacterial inflammations.

One of the first of the NSAIDs was phenylbutazone. This was marvellously effective in acute gout, but it produced a failure of the bone marrow in a very small percentage of patients and for this reason its use has been abandoned. Even if available to you, the risk of using it is too great to justify.

Its next successor was indomethacin and, while this drug does exhibit all of the side-effects common to this class of drug (see below), overall its risk/benefit ratio justifies its continuing use. The reason this class of drug continues to be used is that it is so dramatically effective in acute gout, reducing the pain and inflammation within a few hours. However, the side-effects are a major consideration and are the main limitation on the use of this class of drug.

Damage to the lining membrane of the stomach is so common with non-steroidal anti-inflammatory drug therapy that it can almost be looked upon as an effect of therapy and not merely a side-effect. This effect is usually reversible when therapy is stopped. Changes in the stomach lining are common and many physicians believe that these changes are present in all patients treated with NSAIDs. However, only some patients will develop symptoms, which might include a flare-up of ulcer symptoms, major or minor bleeding from an ulcer, or perforation of a peptic ulcer. Thus, these drugs may aggravate any underlying peptic ulcer disease, even if it is asymptomatic. The use of these drugs increases the risk of complications from a peptic ulcer by three to four times. However, while this risk may seem very high, the overall risk of serious bleeding from the stomach is less than 1 in 300 patients.

Some recently developed NSAIDs, celecoxib (Celebrex) and rofecoxib (Vioxx) and etoricoxib (Arcoxia), have a greatly reduced tendency to adversely affect the lining of the stomach. In these new drugs (the so-called COX-2 inhibitors), the effect of inhibiting the inflammatory prostaglandins in the tissues has been separated from the inhibition of the protective prostaglandins within the stomach. Thus, their undesirable side effect of gastric bleeding has been reduced to an insignificant level, while retaining the analgesic and anti-inflammatory action. However, these drugs have largely been given to patients with osteoarthritis and there are few published reports of their effectiveness in gouty inflammation. One indicates that etori-coxib, administered in a dose of 120 mg once daily is rapidly effective in acute gout and has an effect which is comparable with indomethacin 50 mg taken three times daily. These agents should be of particular value in a patient who has had a previous adverse reaction to NSAIDs which involved the stomach.

The second major side-effect of NSAIDs is on the kidney. Kidney function may deteriorate and control of high blood pressure with anti-hypertensive drugs may be lost. Again, this is usually reversible, particularly if diagnosed and corrected early. This risk is greater in patients with pre-existing renal disease. While it may seem strange to choose to use this drug in patients with pre-existing renal disease, such a choice would be made if this therapy was likely to have fewer risks than other treatments.

Other side-effects of NSAIDs are more troublesome than dangerous, and include headaches and giddiness.

In general, the side-effects of NSAIDs are worse in:

- older patients (over 65 years of age)
- patients with previous gastrointestinal disease
- patients receiving steroids simultaneously
- during the first three months of NSAID therapy
- patients with kidney or liver dysfunction
- patients with heart failure, and
- patients receiving other drug treatments.

In each case, the benefit must be seen to outweigh the risk.

There is no doubt that these drugs are effective in acute gout and that they will usually cause the acute inflammation to subside rapidly. The dose of the drug needed for an acute attack will vary with the severity of the attack, with the individual patient, and with the presence or absence of associated risk factors. A large initial dose will produce a more rapid response but with the potential for a greater risk from side-effects.

Indomethacin, one of the oldest NSAIDs, has been used extensively and is as effective as any of the newer NSAIDs. In a mild attack, a dose of between 25–50 mg (1–2 capsules) is given each eight hours until the acute pain has subsided, when the dose can be reduced and terminated over 4–5 days. It is particularly important to taper the dose off rather than stop it precipitously. In a severe attack, however, the dose could go as high as 50–100 mg each four hours for 24 hours, with rapid reduction to 50 mg three times a day as the acute gout settles, and a further reduction subsequently, with completion after a total of seven days. Such a high dose would only be used in a very severe case of acute gout. Thus, there is the potential for considerable flexibility in dosage and in some patients even one capsule taken at the first sign of acute gout seems to be enough to prevent an acute attack. Thus, the dose needed depends upon the response to be achieved.

Most of the non-steroidal anti-inflammatory drugs are effective within a few hours, provided an adequate dose is taken. In general, the initial dose should be high enough to control inflammation and then the dose and frequency should be steadily but gradually reduced over a period of days. If reduction is too fast, a relapse is likely to occur. Commonly used doses of NSAIDs in an average attack of acute gout are as follows:

- naproxen (Naprosyn): 750 mg initially, followed by 250 mg 8 hourly for 3 days, with gradual subsequent reduction
- sulindac (Clinoril): 400 mg per day in divided doses for 3–4 days, being reduced over the next 3 days
- diclofenac (Voltaren): 50 mg 8 hourly for 48 hours and then 50 mg 12 hourly for 3–4 days
- piroxicam (Feldene): 40 mg a day until relief, when it can be reduced to 20 mg a day until complete subsidence
- ibuprofen (Brufen): 800 mg 8 hourly for 3 days with gradual reduction subsequently, and
- ketoprofen (Orudis): 100 mg 8 hourly, compares with a dose of indomethacin of 50 mg 8 hourly.

There is some evidence that the adverse effect on the stomach is greater with piroxicam. Your medical adviser will have a major role in selecting the most appropriate medication for you.

Summary

- Once the diagnosis of gout has been confirmed, any acute attack should be treated at the earliest possible stage.
- The most appropriate medication will depend upon the likelihood of success as judged by previous responses and the likely side-effects of the various treatments.
- Colchicine is effective in most patients but relief may be delayed for 24 hours and diarrhoea is almost invariable.
- Non-steroidal anti-inflammatory drugs (NSAIDs) are rapidly effective but, except for the COX-2 inhibitors, may irritate the stomach and cause bleeding. They may also interfere with kidney function and the control of raised blood pressure. Other side-effects may limit their usefulness.
- Aspiration of an acute gouty joint may help the inflammation to subside and this may be accelerated by the injection of a corticosteroid into the joint space.
- Full therapy with either colchicine or NSAIDs is preferable to less than full therapy with both, although prophylactic colchicine could be commenced soon after therapy with NSAIDs is begun.
- Always ensure that nothing is done either to raise or to lower the serum urate concentration during treatment for an acute attack of gout. This usually means not altering the medication that was being taken prior to the onset of the acute attack until the attack has settled completely.

eleven

Preventing gout by correcting hyperuricaemia

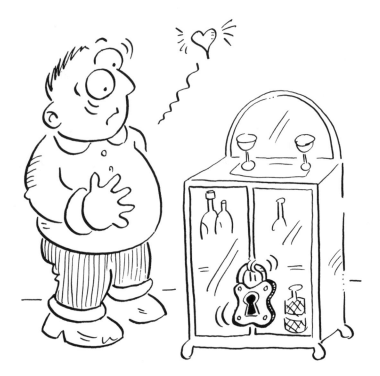

Now that the acute attack of gout has settled completely, what can be done to prevent further acute attacks?

Aims of treatment

While hyperuricaemia persists, the risk of further acute attacks of gout will remain. Thus, preventing acute gout comes down to reducing the serum urate concentration to a normal or 'optimal' level at which the risk of gout is greatly reduced. Only correction of hyperuricaemia will reduce the risk of further acute gout.

It is generally necessary to reduce the serum urate concentration to 0.36 mmol/L (6 mg per 100 mL) or less, if further acute attacks are to be prevented. If, in addition, the gout sufferer has tophi, an even lower serum urate concentration than this (0.30 mmol/L, 5 mg per 100 mL) will probably be needed if the tophi are to dissolve.

How long does the serum urate need to be reduced to this level?

The serum urate needs to be kept within this optimal range permanently. Treatment will be required for as long as the risk of hyperuricaemia persists, i.e. for as long as the cause of the hyperuricaemia remains.

There are only two ways in which hyperuricaemia can be corrected. The first is by finding the cause or causes that can be corrected and correcting them, and the second is by the use of drugs that lower the serum urate. Occasionally, drugs may be useful to reduce the risk of acute attacks temporarily while the patient is undertaking a longer term correction of the cause of the hyperuricaemia, but this is unusual.

Whichever method of reducing the serum urate is chosen, there remains the need for regular observation of the serum urate concentration to ensure that it is below the concentration associated with a risk of acute gout. I would not generally encourage a patient to have the serum urate reduced greatly below this value because sometimes this results in urate from deposits redissolving, and this may increase rather than reduce the risk of acute attacks.

The absence of acute gout is not sufficient guarantee that the serum urate is within the optimal range, so regular measurements of the serum urate are needed until a stable treatment regimen has been developed and shown to be effective. How often the serum urate concentration will need to be measured will therefore vary from patient to patient. More frequent measurements will be needed while the dose of medication is changing, but once a stable dose and a stable urate concentration has been achieved, the serum urate concentration will need to be measured at least every 3 months, or more often if hyperuricaemia persists or control of hyperuricaemia is inadequate or the acute gout recurs.

Correcting factors contributing to hyperuricaemia

The causes of hyperuricaemia have already been considered in chapter 5. Different causes operate in different patients with hyperuricaemia and gout. Some causes, particularly those which are inherited, cannot be corrected by any known modification of lifestyle; these include primary over-production of urate due to a genetic enzyme abnormality or a primary renal under-excretion of urate due to an inherited defect in elimination of urate by the kidney.

There are many mechanisms which will contribute in differing degrees in different patients with gout. While we can identify and sometimes correct contributory factors, this will only correct the underlying hyperuricaemia when those particular factors are making a major contribution to the hyperuricaemia. However, determining the cause and correcting it is the only mechanism whereby a permanent cure of the hyperuricaemia can be achieved and the need for continuing medication eliminated. Correction of the cause is often slow and undramatic and it is difficult for a patient to persist with it unless strongly motivated. Some patients find that they cannot succeed.

There are only a limited number of ways in which permanent correction of hyperuricaemia can be achieved, namely:

- modifying alcohol consumption
- losing excess weight
- modifying diet
- correcting an inadequate urine output
- controlling hypertension
- eliminating drugs causing hyperuricaemia, and
- correcting other diseases which cause hyperuricaemia.

Alcohol

Consumption of alcohol causes hyperuricaemia by both an increase in urate production and a reduction in renal excretion of urate. The binge consumption of alcohol produces a transient and often massive rise in the serum urate concentration with a subsequent fall, and this by itself may precipitate an acute attack of gout. Alcoholic beverages containing yeast (i.e. many beers) also contain purines which are broken down to urate that must be eliminated. In addition, alcohol can contribute to obesity because it contains more kilojoules (calories) than an equivalent weight of sugars and starches (carbohydrates) or protein.

If alcohol consumption is contributing significantly to the hyperuricaemia, reducing or ceasing intake can reduce the serum urate concentration, and sometimes it will fall to a satisfactory range.

The consumption of two standard drinks a day, with more than this at weekends, will probably make a significant contribution to hyperuricaemia (a standard drink contains 10 mL of ethanol, approximately equivalent to 10 oz (300 mL) of beer). However, many people with gout do not consume excessive alcohol and their mild to moderate consumption may not be contributing significantly to their hyperuricaemia.

Body weight

In most Western societies, there is a plentiful supply of food and body weights above that which is optimal for height are common. Often, body weight has increased in the late teens and twenties when vigorous physical activity and sport have been abandoned, but the eating habits developed while physically active are continued. The effect of an increase in body weight beyond the optimal is different in each patient, but in general it will result in both a reduction in the excretion of urate by the kidneys and a moderate increase in urate production. Often it is associated with, and the result of, a past or continuing increase in alcohol consumption. Both high body weight and the alcohol consumption will contribute to the increase of fats in the blood (hypertriglyceridaemia) common in patients who are obese. Loss of even a moderate amount of

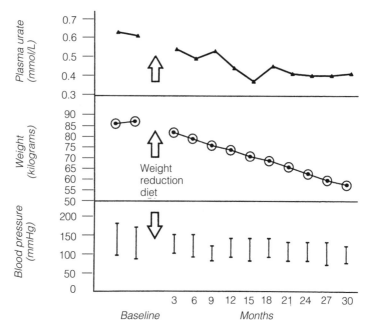

Figure 11.1 Effect of weight reduction on serum urate and systolic blood pressure in a 55-year-old woman who had had two acute attacks of gout.

weight will often result in an improvement in the renal elimination of urate and a fall in urate production, resulting in a
return of the serum urate to an optimal level (figure 11.1).
Hyperlipidaemia will often improve as well.

An old story attributed to Cavershill in 1769 is relevant:

> A certain priest who enjoyed a rich living and had been an old con-
> stant sufferer in gout, happening at last to be taken by the pirates of
> Barbary, was detained there, for the space of two years, a slave, and
> kept constantly at work in the galleys; which had the good effect
> that, afterwards, when he was ransomed from captivity, having lost
> all of his troublesome and monstrous fatness, he never once had a
> fit [of gout], though he lived several years after the event.

Diet

Diet can contribute to hyperuricaemia in several ways. The first
is from the purine content of the diet provided by its cellular
(nuclear) content, partly from any flesh which is consumed and
partly from any rapidly growing plant material. The second refers
to total calorie intake and this includes alcohol consumption and
other factors contributing to an increased body weight.

A very common pattern seen in patients with gout in Australia
is that of a middle-aged male with abdominal obesity who is a
regular consumer of beer, who is 30 per cent above his optimal
weight for height, who consumes meat several times a day and
who also has hypertriglyceridaemia. Correction of such a situation is very difficult because it has arisen as a result of many social
and lifestyle factors. The person's friends and associates often
have a similar lifestyle and any modification of diet and alcohol
consumption is made difficult by social pressures from friends
and by their saying to the patient that lifestyle cannot be important in hyperuricaemia because they do not suffer from gout.
Thus, correction of hyperuricaemia in such patients requires
modification of an established lifestyle pattern, which is extremely difficult for any except the most strongly motivated. Lifestyle
modification to correct the cause of *any* disease is notoriously

difficult to achieve and requires a degree of motivation which can rarely be mustered.

Correction of obesity is made even more difficult by the fact that sufficient kilojoule restriction to cause weight loss may lead to what is referred to as a 'starvation ketosis', i.e. the production of ketone acids during severe kilojoule restriction. Such ketosis may reduce the renal excretion of urate temporarily and aggravate the hyperuricaemia and gout. Thus, if a patient has had more than a few attacks of gout, it is probably wise not to begin any intensive program of weight reduction until the serum urate has been brought into the optimal range, usually by the use of drugs. This may seem contradictory but it is clear that intensive kilojoule restriction can aggravate hyperuricaemia and produce acute gout whereas moderate kilojoule restriction may not.

What is needed is not any crash diet, but a decision on the part of the patient to adopt a healthier lifestyle, with minimal alcohol consumption, sufficient kilojoules to cause a slow weight loss (not exceeding 0.5 kg per week), and moderation of high purine foods. In view of the benefits of lifestyle modification for controlling obesity and hypertriglyceridaemia and the consequent reduction in the risk of heart disease, there is double justification for modification of lifestyle factors. However, rarely can a physician give a patient a more difficult prescription to follow than to suggest that he should lose weight.

Urine volume

A satisfactory rate of urine flow for the kidney to excrete urate is about 1 mL per minute, equivalent to 1440 mL per 24 hours. We have measured the usual rates of urine flow of many healthy young people and find that a surprising proportion (often 30–40 per cent) will pass less than 800–900 mL of urine per 24 hours. An increase in fluid intake to produce a urine flow rate of greater than 1 mL per minute will often facilitate urate excretion by the kidney and cause a modest improvement in the serum urate concentration. Usually this is not great, but it is such a simple manoeuvre that it is worth following, and it benefits overall kidney function as well.

Measurement of the urine flow rate can best be done over a 24-hour period, i.e. all the urine made by the kidneys in the interval between one bladder emptying and another 24 hours later is measured. This is best carried out by emptying the bladder (and discarding that specimen) on arising one morning and then collecting (or measuring the volume of) all urine passed up to and including that passed 24 hours later. Thus, you can easily monitor your own urine volume. It is the final volume of urine which counts, not the volume of fluid ingested. The difference is made up by fluid which is evaporated from the body, which varies from patient to patient and in different climates.

Hypertension

Poorly controlled hypertension can reduce the excretion of urate by the kidney. Correction of this hypertension by one means or another, sometimes involving the use of anti-hypertensive drugs, can benefit the hyperuricaemia, provided the drugs used do not in themselves aggravate the hyperuricaemia.

Drugs retaining urate

The main group of drugs which retain urate are the thiazide or oral diuretics such as chlorothiazide (Chlotride) or frusemide (Lasix). These drugs are used either for the treatment of mild to moderate degrees of hypertension or to correct fluid retention, such as occurs in patients with heart failure.

These drugs go under many different trade names and many anti-hypertensive drugs consist of combinations which include these diuretics, without it being obvious. A patient with gout should check with his/her physician to find out whether their medication contains any of these oral diuretic agents.

While a patient is receiving diuretics, it is very difficult to correct the associated hyperuricaemia. If the hyperuricaemia cannot be corrected otherwise, it may be necessary to review

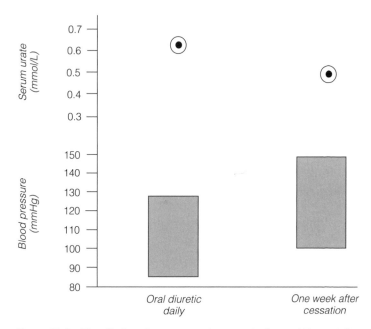

Figure 11.2 The effect on the serum urate concentration and the systolic blood pressure of withdrawing a daily oral diuretic tablet.

the need for the diuretics and to decide whether the same effect can be achieved by the use of other agents (figure 11.2). Sometimes a group of drugs called the ACE inhibitors can have a similar effect to the diuretic drugs without causing the hyperuricaemia. However, sometimes the patient's condition cannot be controlled without diuretic drugs and, when that is so, they must be continued and other approaches attempted to correct the hyperuricaemia.

Other diseases causing hyperuricaemia

There are a few serious medical conditions whose treatment corrects any associated hyperuricaemia. These include hypothyroidism, parathyroid disease and inadequate tissue oxygenation due to a variety of causes, including acidosis due to disease of the lungs and respiratory tract. These all need medical assessment, investigation and, if a disorder is found, treatment. They are all relatively rare contributors to hyperuricaemia, but, if they can be diagnosed and treated, the hyperuricaemia may resolve permanently.

Drug treatment

There are several drugs which can correct hyperuricaemia; these will be considered in detail in the next chapter (chapter 12).

But when should drug therapy be begun? This is usually accepted as being desirable when all of the following situations apply.

- When there is persistent hyperuricaemia, greater than 0.42 mmol/L (7 mg per100 mL)
- When the patient has had 2–3 definite attacks of gout (the interval between early attacks may range between a few months to a couple of years), and
- When the patient is sufficiently persuaded of the need to take tablets regularly and permanently.

Some patients will decide on the need for drug treatment after a single attack of gout, but many patients who start drug treatment before they are fully persuaded will stop treatment once they have been asymptomatic for a period of months or years. However, intermittent treatment to correct hyperuricaemia is not desirable because, unless the cause is corrected, the hyperuricaemia returns and is followed after a time by further gout.

Nobody likes to make decisions about taking tablets for the rest of their lives unless it is absolutely essential. Accordingly, it is generally better not to begin drug treatment to lower the serum urate until you, the patient, are completely persuaded by the frequency and severity of the gout that you need to continue with drug treatment permanently, together with sufficient observation of serum urate to ensure that it stays within the optimal range.

No harm will usually come from delaying treatment to lower the serum urate until there have been several definite attacks of gout, unless you are needing to take drugs such as

NSAIDs frequently to suppress gouty inflammation. In such a situation, severe gout can occur which is often tophaceous and usually difficult to control.

In addition, drug treatment to correct hyperuricaemia should only be begun when the risk of an acute attack of gout is minimal. This means that you should desirably have no acute gout and no residual joint inflammation and should be receiving prophylactic colchicine. Under these conditions, and when any investigation has been completed into contributory factors which might be corrected, drug treatment can begin.

This is probably best undertaken with slowly increasing doses, starting with a low initial dose. This dose can be increased progressively, often with weekly increments, until the optimal dose is reached which can result in appropriate lowering of the serum urate concentration.

As already mentioned, drugs can sometimes be used to control the hyperuricaemia while the cause of the hyperuricaemia is being corrected, if that correction is likely to be prolonged.

How long should drug treatment be continued?

Anyone taking a drug to correct hyperuricaemia should understand that it will need to be continued for as long as the cause of the hyperuricaemia persists or hyperuricaemia is still operating. Usually this will be lifelong.

How is an inadequate response dealt with?

The first evidence of an inadequate response may be a recurrence of the gout. If this occurs while the doses of the drug are increasing in an attempt to achieve optimal urate concentrations, it may be desirable to stop the drug temporarily and recommence it later with increased prophylaxis and more gradual dose increments. On the other hand, if the gout recurs after the serum urate has been normal for some time, it may be best to treat the acute gout in exactly the same way as one would if the serum urate were higher, and to persist with the drug therapy to maintain the normal serum urate.

Acute gout developing during drug treatment requires a very judicious selection and arrangement of drugs and close medical collaboration and supervision in order to control the acute attack of gout at the same time as the serum urate is being lowered to the optimal range.

If the serum urate is not in the optimal range while the patient is taking a standard dose of a urate-lowering drug, the cause needs to be determined and corrected. These causes are very varied. Sometimes, it is as simple as the patient forgetting to take the tablets or forgetting to take the appropriate number of tablets, i.e. taking only two a day instead of three a day, or taking tablets once a day instead of twice a day. Each patient needs to develop a strategy to ensure that the requisite number of tablets is taken on a regular basis. It is always easier to remember to take tablets once a day than more frequently, but even this requires a method of reminding the patient to take the appropriate dose at an appropriate time.

If you are taking the tablets at the appropriate dose on a regular basis, other factors causing the hyperuricaemia need to be sought. These can include excessive consumption of alcohol or drugs which elevate the serum urate, or poorly controlled hypertension. As well, the urate-lowering drug and its dosage may need to be modified.

What needs to be achieved, by one means or another, is a serum urate concentration persistently within the optimal range; if this can be achieved and maintained, recurrences of acute gout will become increasingly fewer until they do not occur at all. Of all chronic diseases, gout is one which should respond to treatment fully and effectively so that further attacks and further complications do not occur. This is the only fully acceptable situation and if it is not achieved, further medical help needs to be sought.

Summary

- Acute gout will usually stop recurring when the serum urate concentration has been returned to optimal values for about twelve months.
- Correction of hyperuricaemia by correction of the causes may be achieved in those patients who are able to correct obesity, regular or excessive alcohol consumption, a high purine diet or a poor urine volume, or when hypertension can be controlled or a diuretic withdrawn. Such corrective measures need to be gradual but sustained.
- When the gout sufferer is persuaded that he/she needs to take medication regularly and permanently to control hyperuricaemia and prevent gout, treatment with a uricosuric drug or a xanthine oxidase inhibitor can be started and an effective dose determined.
- Regular measurement of the serum urate concentration is needed to confirm that the treatment has effectively optimised the serum urate concentration. The absence of acute attacks alone is not sufficient to ensure this since there may be a long interval between acute attacks, even prior to therapy.

twelve

Bringing your urate concentrations down to normal

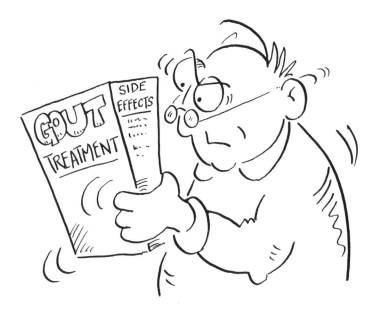

What medication is available?

What are the side-effects?

If, in consultation with your physician, you have decided that the cause of your hyperuricaemia cannot be corrected and that your gout is severe enough to require you to take tablets every day to prevent further attacks, the medication to restore your urate concentration to an optimal level must be chosen.

As with most medication, the benefit to be achieved must be balanced against the risk of developing side-effects. In correcting the hyperuricaemia of gout, there are two alternative and different approaches. Both are valid, both are effective, each has side-effects which are different, and one or other will be better suited to a particular patient with a particular problem. It is a great advantage in correcting hyperuricaemia to have available two different types of medication that act in different ways.

The first group of drugs are the uricosuric agents. These are drugs that increase the excretion of uric acid in the urine. Drugs such as these should be ideal for a patient whose hyperuricaemia is caused by a reduced excretion of uric acid in the urine.

The second major group of drugs are xanthine oxidase inhibitors. The only drug in this class currently available is allopurinol, which acts to reduce the amount of urate produced by the body and is most useful in patients who are either over-producing urate or who are consuming large amounts of purines.

However, as already indicated, not all patients fit easily into a category of either over-producers or under-excretors of urate, and many have features of both. However, if it is possible to define the major contribution to the hyperuricaemia in a particular patient, an appropriate drug can be selected to correct this. The likelihood of side-effects from one particular agent may dominate the choice of drugs to use.

Uricosuric drugs

Uricosuric drugs increase the urinary excretion of uric acid. They act on the uric acid transport mechanisms in the kidney

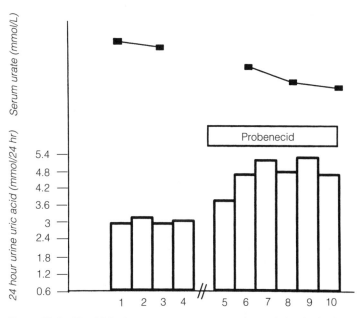

Figure 12.1 The fall in the serum urate concentration and the rise in the urinary urate excretion with the administration of increasing doses of probenecid.

tubule to increase the amount of uric acid which is excreted in the urine. This means they increase the 24-hour excretion of uric acid in the urine.

The serum urate concentration at any particular time is a balance between the urate produced in the body and the urate which is eliminated (two-thirds of which is eliminated by the kidney). Thus, in a state where urate production is stable, an increase in the excretion of urate by the kidney will lower the serum urate concentration in the blood (figure 12.1). Such a drug is ideal for a person with a low urinary excretion of urate, a so-called under-excretor of urate, with a low urate clearance and a low 24-hour urine urate excretion.

The price of restoring the serum urate toward a more optimal range by this means is an increase in the uric acid concentration in the urine. As uric acid is relatively insoluble in the urine, particularly if that urine is concentrated or very acidic, an increase in the concentration of uric acid in the urine might lead to crystallisation of uric acid within the kidney or urinary tract (crystalluria). The actual risk of crystallisation within the renal tract will depend upon both the concentration of uric acid in the urine and its acidity.

The increase in the urinary uric acid is much higher during the first few weeks of treatment with a uricosuric drug and, during this time, the risk of crystalluria is usually controlled by ensuring that the patient has a dilute urine (by increasing fluid consumption) and by reducing acidity or alkalinising the urine (often by administering sodium bicarbonate in a dose of between 3 and 6 g per 24 hours, sufficient to turn litmus paper moistened with urine from pink to blue). After a few weeks, the large increase in urinary uric acid excretion falls back to a value only a little above that before the uricosuric drug was administered, and the risk of uric acid crystalluria and stone formation is much less. Nonetheless, during this time it is important to maintain a high urine flow rate (diuresis)—in fact, any person taking a uricosuric drug should ensure that he or she is always able to maintain a good urine volume.

Uric acid crystalluria may be particularly troublesome when starting treatment (and this applies to re-starting after having stopped treatment), or if the urine is very concentrated, as occurs following a period of limited fluid intake or excessive fluid loss (for example in hot weather). Particularly in an aeroplane flight, the urine may become increasingly concentrated.

I have referred to the hazard of uric acid crystalluria, both here and in previous chapters. A high uric acid concentration in a concentrated or acid urine can allow crystals of uric acid to deposit either within the collecting ducts of the kidney or within the renal pelvis and ureter. Crystals in the collecting ducts may impair the function of the kidney (although this may be relieved by an alkaline diuresis); in the kidney pelvis or ureter they may cause the formation of gravel or a kidney stone, and may cause either the severe pain of renal colic or blood in the urine.

Thus, successful therapy with a uricosuric drug requires a sufficient urine flow (preferably a minimum of 2 litres per 24 hours), the absence of any past history of a renal calculus or stone, and renal function which is at least half of the normal. Any acute deterioration of renal function needs to be treated with an alkaline diuresis (bicarbonate and increased fluid volume), which will often reverse the deterioration of renal function effectively.

The effect on the serum urate of a uricosuric drug is usually dose-related, increasing with an increasing dose of the drug. However, the response is reduced if kidney disease is present and there may be no detectable response if renal function is less than half normal. Again, the aim of treatment is to restore the serum urate to an optimal level (0.36 mmol/L or 6 mg per 100 mL) and unless this can be achieved, the treatment is not achieving the goal and needs to be reviewed.

I have referred to the importance of minimising the risk of acute attacks of gout by making any changes in the serum urate gradual rather than abrupt. Sometimes, a full dose of a uricosuric drug can lower the serum urate so rapidly that an acute attack of gout may occur. This risk is reduced if the dose of the urate-lowering drug is increased gradually; the resulting gradual but definite fall in the serum urate concentration rarely brings on an acute attack of gout. There is rarely any need to lower the serum urate rapidly.

Types of uricosuric drugs

Probenecid (Benemid, Procid)

This drug, discovered in 1950, was the first to be used to correct hyperuricaemia. At that time there was great excitement that a drug was now available which could correct hyperuricaemia, thereby preventing acute attacks of gout and causing resorption of tophi. That gout is still occurring almost 50 years later indicates that it is not lack of available therapy which allows the disease to be perpetuated and that the greater difficulty is ensuring that the right medication is taken by the right person at the right time.

Probenecid has multiple effects on membranes in the body and, within the kidney, it also blocks the excretion of penicillin and penicillin derivatives, aspirin, and several other drugs including dapsone. Thus, when probenecid is given to a patient who is also receiving penicillin, the blood level of penicillin will be much higher than without the probenecid. This is exactly the opposite of its effect on uric acid, where it reduces the blood level and increases the urine concentration. This illustrates the fact that drugs may affect multiple organs and may act at different sites within the body. Aspirin can neutralise the uricosuric effect of probenecid.

Probenecid needs to be given 2 or 3 times a day, the dose usually being one tablet of 500 mg which is taken each 8–12 hours. Since few people can manage to take tablets 8 hourly on a long-term basis, in practice probenecid is usually taken twice daily. A serum urate of less than 0.36 mmol/L will be achieved in 60 per cent of patients taking 1 g of probenecid per day and in 85 per cent of patients taking 2 g of probenecid per day. However, for one reason or another, up to 25 per cent of patients do not achieve adequate control of their serum urate with this drug.

The side-effects from probenecid are rarely serious and are often in the form of nausea or a rash, which may occur in up to 10 per cent of patients. The risk from the high urine uric acid remains and the patient taking this drug needs to be constantly aware of the importance of a good urine flow rate. The urine is usually alkalinized with sodium bicarbonate capsules by mouth during the first weeks of uricosuric therapy when the uric acid concentration in the urine is highest. It thereby reduces the risk of uric acid crystal formation and the formation of uric acid calculi (stones).

Sulfinpyrazone (Anturan)

On a weight-for-weight basis, this drug is more potent than probenecid (100 mg of sulfinpyrazone will have a uricosuric effect similar to 500 mg of probenecid). It has the additional benefit of an improvement in platelet survival and a reduction of platelet stickiness, which is beneficial in preventing blood clots forming within the vascular system. However, it has recently been withdrawn from use throughout the world.

Other uricosuric drugs

Aspirin, in a sufficient dose, increases the excretion of uric acid in the urine. It achieves this by the presence of one of its breakdown products, salicylate, within the fluid in the renal tubules. The amount of salicylate can be increased by alkalinising the urine. However, most patients will need a dose of 5 g of aspirin and 5 g of sodium bicarbonate each day to achieve an effective uricosuric response. This amounts to 15 tablets of aspirin in a day spread over 3 or 4 doses. Such frequent treatment is rarely practical. It is, nonetheless, an interesting observation which may occasionally be useful in therapy.

Diflunisal, which is related to aspirin, has both uricosuric and anti-inflammatory properties and may be useful in a patient who develops acute gout each time urate-lowering therapy is begun. Its urate lowering potential is slightly less than that of allopurinol but it may be a useful alternative drug.

Another drug, benzbromarone, is a potent uricosuric drug but is not available in some countries. Similarly, azapropazone has both anti-inflammatory and urate-lowering potential but it too is not available in many countries and would be used only when standard treatment is not effective.

A newly developed anti-hypertensive agent, losarton, which is an antagonist to the angiotensin II receptor, has been shown also to have a modest uricosuric action. This might be useful in a patient whose urate response to drugs is otherwise inadequate.

Allopurinol

Zyloprim, Progout, Zygout, Capurate

Allopurinol inhibits an enzyme which is required for the final step in the production of uric acid. Inhibition of this enzyme, xanthine oxidase, therefore reduces the amount of uric acid produced within the body, although it slightly increases the amount of the uric acid precursors hypoxanthine and xanthine. It reduces urate and purine production overall so that the total production of purines, including uric acid and its precursors, is lowered. As a consequence, the total excretion of uric acid, xanthine and hypoxanthine is reduced (figure 12.2). This is desirable as far as uric acid is concerned. However, xanthine is even less soluble than uric acid and there is a potential for crystallisation of xanthine from the urine. In practice, this rarely occurs (except in the very rare genetic over-producers of uric acid). The risk of crystallisation within the renal tract is reduced because the total purine excretion is distributed through three compounds rather than one (uric acid) and the risk of crystallisation of each of these substances is independent of the presence of the other.

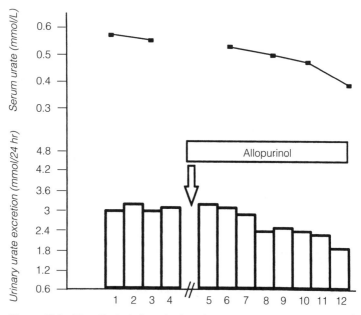

Figure 12.2 The effect of allopurinol on the serum urate concentration and the urinary urate excretion.

Allopurinol itself is broken down in the body to another drug called oxypurinol, which is its active form. Allopurinol is the form in which it is taken because oxypurinol is not well absorbed from the stomach. The conversion occurs rapidly, so allopurinol can only be detected for a few hours after taking a tablet, whereas oxypurinol can be shown to be present for more than 24 hours after a tablet of allopurinol has been taken. Thus it is the oxypurinol which is inhibiting the xanthine oxidase.

Interestingly, it is the enzyme which is inhibited, xanthine oxidase, that converts the allopurinol to oxypurinol. The xanthine oxidase is only partially blocked, so adequate concentrations of oxypurinol are maintained. Even after a single dose, it takes over seven days for oxypurinol to disappear from the body. Because oxypurinol remains in the body for such a long period, once-daily therapy is possible—this is a distinct advantage in a condition where treatment will need to be continued for many years.

Given these mechanisms of action, allopurinol should be ideal treatment for any situation where there is excessive production of uric acid. Accordingly, it is as useful in primary (genetic) over-production of urate as it is in over-consumption of purines or following cancer chemotherapy (which causes cellular breakdown and excessive production of uric acid). The only cloud on its horizon is its side-effects, which will be dealt with later.

Allopurinol comes in tablets of 100 mg or 300 mg. As with all drugs to lower the serum urate, alteration of the serum urate should be slow and dosage should begin at a low dose and should increase gradually. Thus, an initial dose might be 50–100 mg per day and this can be increased slowly, usually at weekly intervals, until a total dose of 300–400 mg per day is being taken. Eight-five per cent of patients will have a normal serum urate when taking 300 mg per day, although some may have a satisfactory serum urate on a somewhat lower dose than this. Occasional large patients may need more than 300 mg per day but rarely should there be a need for more than 400 mg per day unless another factor is operating to limit the response. If the serum urate is not optimal at a dose of 400 mg per day, alternative causes for hyperuricaemia need to be sought and corrected in their own right. This could apply, for instance, to the concurrent administration of a diuretic drug.

Occasionally, a uricosuric drug is given at the same time as allopurinol, usually in the hope of lowering the serum urate further. This has a complicated effect. The uricosuric drug will have some uricosuric effect, the degree depending upon the dose given and the responsiveness of the kidney. However, it will also increase the kidney excretion of the active metabolite of allopurinol, oxypurinol, and this will lower the concentration of oxypurinol and thereby reduce its urate-lowering effect. The overall effect will depend upon the balance between these two processes operating in different directions. It may occasionally be desirable to use these drugs together but it is a complex treatment which should be used infrequently and with close observation of its effect.

The effect of kidney disease on the dose of allopurinol also needs to be considered. Since the active metabolite of allopurinol, oxypurinol, is principally excreted by the kidney, its excretion is reduced in the presence of kidney disease. Therefore, unless the dose is reduced in proportion to renal function, the concentration of oxypurinol in the tissues may be excessive. There has been some evidence to suggest that side-effects, particularly hypersensitivity, are greater in patients with a high serum concentration of oxypurinol. Therefore, if a patient has two-thirds of normal renal function, the dose of allopurinol might be reduced to two-thirds of the usual, namely 200 mg per day, whereas if renal function is one-third of normal, the usual dose might be only 100 mg per day. However, efficacy of therapy depends on the serum urate concentration and this may need to be used as a guide to dosage. If hyperuricaemia persists, other causes for the hyperuricaemia need to be corrected instead of increasing the dose of allopurinol out of proportion to the patient's renal function.

Two other uncommon drugs, azathioprine (Imuran, used as an immunosuppressant in tissue transplantation) and 6-mercaptopurine (used in certain cancers of the bone marrow) are normally metabolised by xanthine oxidase. Accordingly, their effect is greatly increased by the concurrent administration of allopurinol and their dose needs to be reduced accordingly, usually to about a quarter of what it would be without the allopurinol. Use of either of these drugs with allopurinol is uncommon but, unless the dose is reduced, severe suppression of the bone marrow can occur.

Allopurinol treatment is also very effective against kidney stones, either of uric acid or calcium oxalate. Its value in treating renal stones is not necessarily related to the urate concentration in the blood.

Side-effects of allopurinol

About 2 per cent of patients taking allopurinol will develop an allergic rash with the drug which will usually subside on withdrawal of the drug. Sometimes, the rash does not recur when the allopurinol is given at a slightly lower dose, although this lower dose may be less effective in controlling the hyperuricaemia.

Other side-effects, commonly referred to as a general hypersensitivity, are much more serious and may even be life-threatening. These often include fever, dermatitis (with loss of superficial skin), liver disease, and inflammation of the kidney with rapid deterioration of kidney function. This hypersensitivity reaction may come on suddenly and be unpredictable. It can occur with other drugs and will often subside more rapidly if treated with prednisone.

Which patients are likely to develop this side-effect cannot be predicted in advance, although there is some suggestion (which is not universally accepted) that the risk is greater if the dose of allopurinol is high or if the patient has renal disease or is taking diuretics. One needs to remember that allopurinol's effectiveness in the presence of renal disease is one of its advantages. Still, the risk is small and serious hypersensitivity reactions occur in less than one in 10 000 patients taking allopurinol. The risk is slightly increased if the patient is taking the antibiotic ampicillin at the same time.

As with other allergic states, desensitisation to the drug may be undertaken for minor allergic side-effects, such as an itchy rash, although it is rarely undertaken and rarely successful for major sensitisation which involves kidney or liver disorder, with a fever. The success of desensitisation is unpredictable and it may be hazardous if the underlying hypersensitivity reaction was serious or life-threatening.

This puts into perspective my earlier comment that the use of a drug or medication is a balance between the good it does and the harm it may do. In most cases, the good outweighs the harm, but some potential for harm is always present with any effective medication and this harm will vary with the drug and with the individual patient. Thus a gout patient with renal disease would respond less well to a uricosuric drug, making allopurinol the drug of choice with the dose adjusted to renal function, but there is a slightly increased risk of drug hypersensitivity. In a patient with a known history of allopurinol hypersensitivity, a uricosuric drug would usually be needed. However, if that patient had previously had renal colic from a renal calculus, there would need to be great caution in the administration of a uricosuric drug: to reduce the risk of further uric acid crystal and renal calculus formation it should be given only if the patient could consistently maintain a urine volume of at least 2500 mL per 24 hours and if that urine could be kept slightly alkaline with sodium bicarbonate.

Role of the diet in gout in patients treated with urate lowering drugs

As discussed, we see the diet as a possible contributor to, rather than a major cause of, a high urate concentration and gout. The hyperuricaemia, if prolonged and sufficiently elevated, can contribute to the development and continuation of the gout but this contribution will become less as a lower serum urate is maintained. In patients whose serum urate is persistently less than 0.30 mmols/l (5 mg/100 ml), while on treatment with urate lowering drugs, there should be no need for any additional modification to diet, except for the avoidance of binge eating and drinking and the maintenance of an optimal body weight.

How then can the diet contribute to hyperuricaemia?

Those who consume large quantities of purine containing foods will exhibit an increased production of uric acid when these dietary purines are broken down in the body, as shown in table 5.1. The consumption of a large quantity of a food low in purines can lead to the production of more purines than the consumption of a small amount of a high purine containing food. Thus the amount of the food consumed is as important as its relative purine content. Foods that are relatively high in purines, which most people are able to omit from their diet, are shown in table 12.1. It is reasonable to include one moderate sized serving of meat or fish each day.

Alcohol causes an increase in the production of uric acid and other purines and also reduces the elimination of uric acid in the urine. This is particularly severe in binge drinking, and quite severe hyperuricaemia can occur after an alcoholic binge. The diet can therefore result in hyperuricaemia from the purine content of the foods consumed, as well as from the altered metabolism resulting from excessive alcohol consumption.

Energy resulting from an imbalance of kilojoule (calorie) intake relative to energy utilisation results in storage of this energy as fat and, if sufficiently prolonged, this can result in obesity. Such obesity can lead to insulin resistance, which promotes hyperuricaemia by a reduction in urate excretion. Weight loss improves insulin resistance, and this allows more urate to be eliminated by the kidney, thus lowering the serum urate.

Table 12.1

Foods relatively high in purines which contribute to hyperuricaemia and which can readily be reduced or eliminated from diet

Anchovies, herring, sardines, scallops, lobster, shellfish
Asparagus, mushrooms, cauliflower
Kidneys, liver, sweetbreads, game meats
Beans, peas, lentils, sprouts

Too small a fluid intake can contribute to hyperuricaemia. The minimum urine volume should be two litres per day, but larger volumes are beneficial.

It is important, however, to recognise that individual patients with gout have different factors contributing to the development of hyperuricaemia.

Certain dietary constituents are thought to precipitate acute attacks of gout in particular susceptible subjects. Red wine is reputed to be one, and many patients with gout have noticed this and believe this to be so from their personal experience. Such susceptibility is very individual, and most individuals with gout will inevitably seek to identify dietary precipitants of their acute attacks. These vary so widely that it is not possible to list them all. However, each gout sufferer will need to make his or her own list and learn to avoid those precipitating factors.

Paradoxically, **severe** kilojoule (calorie) restriction can aggravate hyperuricaemia because of the formation of ketone bodies, which reduce the excretion of urate by the kidney. Anyone who has recently suffered from acute gout should not aim to reduce the serum urate too rapidly nor should they at any time aim to lose more than half a kilogram of weight per week. Weight control is particularly to be desired and abdominal girth kept to less than 100 cm (40 inches).

Any diet that is taken for a medical condition needs to be lifelong and must be permanently acceptable to the patient. A person can rarely accept the total elimination from their diet of a much-loved dietary constituent. However, considerable modification and restriction of the amount consumed is generally more tolerable. This is why the best diet for someone with gout is a balanced one in which all food types (except high purine foods) are taken in moderation. Such a prudent diet is recommended by national heart foundations in various countries. This is beneficial for any associated cardiovascular complications of gout, as well as in the attempt to minimise any tendency to hyperuricaemia from dietary constituents. An example of a diet which can be taken permanently and not aggravate hyperuricaemia is shown in table 12.2. Meals need to be sufficiently varied so that they are still tasty and satisfying.

Table 12.2

Example of a low purine diet

Breakfast:	Cereal, milk (reduced fat preferable)
	Fruit
	Toast, margarine, marmalade, jam
	Egg if desired
	Tea or coffee
Lunch:	Salad of lettuce, tomato, beetroot, pineapple, carrot, cheese, oil and vinegar dressing
	Bread, margarine, pasta dishes
	Fruit
	Tea or coffee
Dinner:	Meat or fish (100g) purine containing
	Low purine vegetables, potato, pumpkin, cabbage
	Fruit, ice cream
	Tea or coffee

Aim for a fluid intake of three litres per 24 hours. This could consist of unsweetened tea or coffee, low-calorie drinks and water. Alcohol best kept to a minimum. Snacks between meals to consist of liquids as above, plus fruit.

It is also notable that, if a patient's serum urate is within the recommended range (less than 0.36 mmol/L or 6 mg/100 ml), this should be sufficient to control any tendency to acute gout without the need for dietary modification to lower the serum urate further. If, however, the drugs to lower serum urate have not brought the serum urate to this recommended level, dietary restriction of purines may sometimes be needed. However, it will only have a minor contribution to the control of hyperuricaemia, and review of the dosage of the urate lowering drugs will probably be needed.

Summary

- Medications to optimise serum urate concentrations may either be uricosuric (promote renal excretion of urate) or inhibitors of xanthine oxidase (reduce urate production). Each has a different action and side-effects.

- The choice of therapy is often determined by the likely side-effects.
- As well as lowering serum urate concentrations, uricosuric drugs increase the concentration of urate in the urine with the potential for uric acid crystalluria if the urine becomes concentrated or acidic. This is prevented by keeping the urine dilute and alkaline, but the risk recurs each time the urine becomes concentrated or the medication is stopped and started.
- The precipitation of acute attacks of gout by abrupt changes in urate concentrations can be minimised by increasing the dose of urate-lowering medications gradually.
- Probenecid in a dose of 1 gram/day will optimise the serum urate in 60% of patients and 2 grams/day will achieve this in 85% of patients. Sulfinpyrazone is similarly effective in a dose of 200 mg twice daily.
- Allopurinol, a chemical structurally similar to the purine bases, is changed within the body to oxypurinol, its active principle, which acts for over 24 hours. Eighty-five per cent of patients achieve a normal serum urate on 300 mg of allopurinol per day.
- The most serious side-effect of allopurinol is a hypersensitivity which may occur unpredictably in a frequency of less than 1 in 10 000 patients. Its severity ranges from a transient rash to a life-endangering illness with severe dermatitis and skin loss, fever, and reduced function of the liver and kidneys. Occasionally desensitisation to the drug is possible.

thirteen

Questions and answers about gout

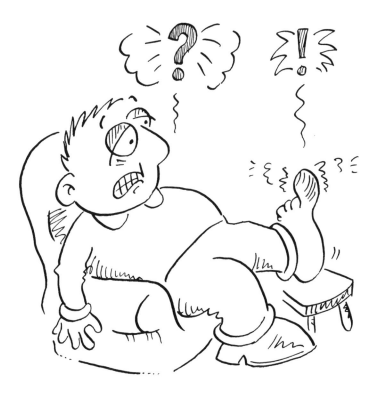

This chapter brings together specific answers to some common questions for your convenience.

What are the basic causes of the high uric acid concentration in gout?

Popular ideas about gout commonly blame the gout on the sufferer's diet or alcohol consumption or obesity. This book has sought to make it clear that the factors contributing to gout are many and that the different causes operate in different degrees in different patients. In each patient, several factors are probably operating at once and these ultimately cause the development of an increased concentration of urate in the body tissues; if this is sustained for a sufficient period, it can lead to urate crystal precipitation and the acute inflammatory response to this which we call an acute attack of gout.

Thus, in some patients, the cause of their hyperuricaemia may be principally environmental (lifestyle) factors involving over-nutrition and excessive alcohol consumption. There are others in whom the gout is totally due to genetic factors and environmental factors have no role. In many other patients, there is a combination of both environmental factors (such as over-nutrition and over-consumption of alcohol) and genetic factors (poor renal excretory capacity for urate). Thus, acute gout is a symptom complex with many causes, all of which lead to urate crystal deposition, and the same clinical pattern may occur no matter what the cause of the elevated urate concentration. Thus, some patients with hyperuricaemia and gout will be thin and may never take any alcohol and yet have severe hyperuricaemia—their gout is due primarily to genetic factors and is not modified by altering the diet. Others may be obese and take alcohol regularly and may never develop hyperuricaemia and gout—these fortunate few are born with kidneys able to eliminate a substantial urate load without any elevation of the urate concentration in the blood.

These very basic facts need to be kept in mind.

What effect does alcohol have on gout, and is there any one alcoholic drink which is better or worse than others as far as gout is concerned?

To answer this, we need to sort out two effects. The first is the effect which works via the urate concentration, which depends on the alcohol content, and the second relates to the particular alcoholic beverage consumed and not to the alcohol it contains.

The effect of specific alcoholic drinks depends on both their alcohol content and their purine content. The only alcoholic drink which contains significant amounts of purine is beer (this comes from its yeast content) and these purines are broken down in the body to urate.

Alcohol increases the body's production of urate and reduces the kidneys' excretion of urate. Thus, there is a high correlation between the amount of alcohol consumed and the average level of serum urate concentration. The consumption of as little as 20 mL of ethanol (two standard drinks) a day is sufficient to have a significant effect upon the serum urate concentration. This would be provided by 500 mL or 20 oz of regular beer (one large bottle usually contains 740 mL or 26 oz). Light beer contains less alcohol than heavy or regular beer and will accordingly have less effect on the serum urate concentration. In addition, alcohol, on a weight for weight basis, contains almost twice as many kilojoules per gram as sugar. Thus, the energy from alcohol consumption is more difficult to utilise and tends to cause obesity, so that the problems and effect of obesity on the serum urate are added to those of alcohol.

Fluctuations in the serum urate can often precipitate acute attacks and wide fluctuations in serum urate can result from indiscretions or excesses of food and alcohol, particularly of alcohol because alcoholic binge drinking is not uncommon in many communities. Binge drinking can therefore lead to severe, though short-lived, elevations of the serum urate concentration and these rises can sometimes precipitate acute attacks.

Although the mechanisms involved are complex, there is no doubt that alcohol consumption, particularly if it is regular and of more than mild degree, can both cause hyperuricaemia as well as precipitate acute attacks of gout.

It is commonly believed that red wine is worse than white wine in causing an acute attack of gout. However, there has been no scientific study to establish this and there are so many factors which can precipitate an acute attack of gout in a person with severe hyperuricaemia that it would be very difficult to prove that one alcoholic beverage was worse than another in provoking acute attacks. What is clear is that once the serum urate has been restored to normal, neither red wine nor white wine in moderation should precipitate an acute attack of gout. The message is that individual sensitivity may well exist, and if you have a suspicion that a particular beverage such as red wine precipitates your acute gout, then it is best to avoid it until your serum urate is completely normal. If it continues to be a problem then, avoidance must continue.

What does body weight have to do with gout?

In almost all populations throughout the world there is a high correlation between body weight and the serum urate concentration, so that the higher the body weight, the greater the serum urate concentration. One measure of body weight and of obesity is called the body mass index (BMI), which is calculated by dividing the body weight in kilograms by the square of the height in metres. If this exceeds 27.5, the subject can be regarded as obese. Perhaps more simply, a weight of 30 per cent above the desirable weight for height can be regarded as greater than optimal. More recently, it has been suggested that an abdominal girth at the waist exceeding 102 cm in men or 88 cm in women is a simple indicator of obesity. Another important contributor seems to be excessive weight gain in young adulthood.

In particular individuals, loss of weight leads to a fall in the serum urate concentration due to three factors:

• an increased excretion of urate by the kidney
• a reduction in the amount of urate produced within the body, and

- a fall in blood pressure, which again facilitates renal excretion of urate.

Beneficial effects on the serum urate from weight reduction can often be seen with even minor weight loss in some patients, and it is to be expected that an individual who loses weight will have a corresponding fall in the serum urate concentration. Thus, it appears that there is a cause and effect relationship between body weight and serum urate concentration.

Hyperuricaemia is very common in sumo wrestlers in Japan. These men consume in excess of 1200 kilojoules per day (more than 50 per cent above the usual) and develop obesity and hypertriglyceridaemia as well as hyperuricaemia. They also have a higher than average incidence of hypertension and diabetes. Thus, in some ways, they are a model of our patient with gout who develops hyperuricaemia because of overnutrition. Such overnutrition can occur because of excessive consumption of kilojoules in the form of either food or beverages.

A little needs to be said about the problem of obesity in industrialised and Westernised societies, where people may well feel that most members of their society are healthy rather than obese. Using strictly medical criteria of health, obese subjects (as defined by the criteria above) are very common in many communities and the health problems from this degree of overweight do not develop until mid to later life. The reason for this obesity in many Westernised communities is a mismatch between food intake and energy output. Animals expend a minimum amount of energy to take in a maximum amount of food. While this works well in the wild, where the animal has to seek food, the two activities of collecting and consuming have become separated in industrialised societies. Most of these societies can be classed as opulent as far as food availability is concerned and there are major societal pressures to consume food, much of which contains fat; and fat, like alcohol, is very high in kilojoules on a weight basis. Most social interactions in a Western society involve the consumption of food. In addition, overeating has often become a response to stress. If this excessive kilojoule consumption were compensated by an increase in exercise, there would be little problem in energy balance, but exercise is time-consuming and only a relatively small proportion of the population exercise effectively. Thus, obesity is a major health problem in Western industrialised societies and, in some people, the factors which lead to obesity also lead to hyperuricaemia. Having said all this, it is important to recognise that there are inherited or genetic, as well as environmental, factors involved in obesity and that these are being increasingly well identified. A person with a genetic susceptibility to obesity will have more difficulty in adapting to a high kilojoule diet than another. In such a person, kilojoule restriction may do little to achieve weight loss. Fortunately, progress is being made with this problem and, if this continues, great advances in the control of obesity will result.

How important is one's diet in the development of gout?

There may be some dietary constituents which will precipitate an acute attack of gout in a hyperuricaemic individual. These tend to be individual peculiarities and there is no predictable pattern in such food consumption. Specific foods which precipitate gout in an individual (such as prawns) should be avoided but there is no way of selecting these in advance. They can only be learnt by experience. It is not a problem if the serum urate is normal.

Diet would have its main effect on gout by its effect on the serum urate concentration. The major dietary factors having an effect on the serum urate concentration are:

- body weight
- alcohol consumption
- dietary purines, and
- fluid consumption.

Effect of body weight

An imbalance between urate production and excretion as an effect of overnutrition has already been discussed and, insofar as the diet contributes to this overnutrition, the total kilojoule consumption of the diet will contribute to the hyperuricaemia.

Alcohol consumption

As already indicated, alcohol (regarded as part of the diet) increases urate production and reduces urate excretion because of its breakdown to lactate. It may also contain purines. Accordingly, regular alcohol consumption may contribute significantly to hyperuricaemia.

Dietary purines

If the intake of foods which are degraded to uric acid produces more uric acid than can be eliminated by the body, hyperuricaemia can result. Tissues being broken down to produce uric acid are those containing nuclei, particularly all flesh (whether red or white, meat or fish, table 5.2). In those who consume excessive purines, but whose kidneys are able to eliminate such a urate load, the serum concentration of urate may remain normal. However, in these people there may be a very high urine concentration of urate which can cause problems in the form of renal stones made of uric acid or calcium oxalate.

Fluid consumption

The kidney needs to produce a urine flow of at least 1500 mL a day to eliminate the uric acid produced in that time. Those who pass a smaller urine volume than this may have an increase in their serum urate because their renal elimination is less than it should be.

Diet in controlled gout

Most importantly, however, in subjects with gout whose serum urate has been returned to normal by treatment, the diet will generally have a minimal effect on their gout provided there are no excesses of alcohol or food which can cause rapid fluctuations in an elevated serum urate concentration.

What effect will my gout have on my life expectancy?

If your serum urate concentration is normal (even if this has been achieved by the use of urate-lowering drugs) your gout will, in itself, have no effect upon your life expectancy. I said 'in itself', and this is important because the effect will depend upon the cause of the gout and the effect of that cause on your life expectancy. One's life expectancy depends chiefly upon the health of one's blood vessels, particularly the blood vessels to the heart, the brain and the kidneys. This means that factors that cause blood vessel disease (atherosclerosis) can reduce life expectancy, and some of these can also give rise to hyperuricaemia. If you merely correct the hyperuricaemia and allow the other factors causing the vascular disease to persist, life expectancy will not be helped by the correction of the hyperuricaemia and gout. Thus, life expectancy is known to be reduced in the presence of obesity, hypertension, elevated blood fats (such as cholesterol or triglycerides), kidney disease, or heart disease needing treatment with diuretic drugs. These can all lead to an increased risk of vascular disease as well as to hyperuricaemia.

If you want a long and healthy life, concentrate on the vascular risk factors as listed and the hyperuricaemia will probably look after itself. Your life expectancy will depend more upon the associated diseases, particularly of the blood vessels, than on the gout.

Should the management of gout be different in the elderly?

The same principles apply to the management of gout at any age. However, this refers to the biological age, or tissue age, rather than the chronological age. (Some people aged 70 are much healthier and have fewer signs of ageing than other patients aged 60.) This consideration, and the presence of other associated diseases, may indicate the need for some modification of treatment goals. In addition, the presence of other associated diseases may limit the intensity with which normalisation of the serum urate should be pursued. If normalisation can be achieved simply, then it is desirable. This said, if its achievement produces major difficulties, it may be better to rely more on symptomatic treatment of the gout rather than to undertake heroic measures to control the hyperuricaemia. However, if a normal urate concentration can be achieved, it is as desirable in the elderly as in the younger age group.

What are the greatest current problems in the management of gout?

One of the biggest problems in managing hyperuricaemia is the patient who develops sensitivity to the drugs that need to be used. This is particularly so if the drug is allopurinol, although the frequency of severe sensitivity is probably less than 1 in 10 000 patients treated. Sensitivity to allopurinol can show up either as an allergic skin reaction or as a serious multisystem illness. It also makes a very useful drug unavailable for further use. The severity of the problem then depends upon whether an alternative drug can be effective in the particular patient.

A second major problem is the patient who is dependent upon large doses of oral diuretics such as chlorothiazide or frusemide for another condition such as heart failure. If these drugs cannot be reduced or withdrawn, it may be very difficult to correct the resulting hyperuricaemia. Best of all would be to correct the condition which causes the need for the diuretic drugs to be administered.

The third common problem is the patient whose serum urate remains elevated despite an apparently adequate dose of the urate lowering drug. This can be a major problem in management and can occur when the original cause of the hyperuricaemia is persisting. It can tax the ingenuity of the most able physician.

The fourth current problem is the patient who develops acute attacks of gout but is intolerant of non-steroidal anti-inflammatory drugs or other treatments for his acute gout. The problem is particularly acute in such patients who develop an acute attack each time therapy aimed at bringing the serum urate to an optimal value is commenced.

Since we know how to treat gout, why are people still suffering from acute gout?

The first answer to this relates to the difficulty of modifying lifestyle factors (including obesity, diet and alcohol consumption) which contribute so frequently to the hyperuricaemia. Many patients find it difficult to correct the causative factors for their hyperuricaemia.

However, there are still difficulties in persuading people to take the necessary medication to control their hyperuricaemia and gout. There is a real problem for many people in remembering to take tablets on a regular basis for a condition which produces symptoms only intermittently. Remembering to take tablets is easier if they are able to be taken once a day rather than twice a day; if medication is effective taken daily rather than each 8–12 hours, compliance by regular consumption is improved.

A second problem is that patients who take urate-lowering tablets regularly tend to be discouraged when an acute attack of gout occurs despite the tablets. They do not realise that the serum urate needs to be within the normal range for at least a year before the frequency of acute attacks will become less and the attacks will ultimately disappear.

The third problem is for the patient to know which tablet to take and when. Although most gout sufferers have this knowledge, it is clearly not universal.

One of the aims of this book is that knowledge and understanding of the treatment of this condition will improve to the extent that gout will become an uncommon disease. Throughout, I have emphasised that patient knowledge and understanding about the disease is vital for effective management of a chronic condition which has long asymptomatic intervals, and it is a cooperative effort between the patient and the patient's medical attendant which can lead most effectively to the elimination of gout as a health problem.

Index